ARE THO
1952. A do
has also studied anthroposophic medicine,
homeopathy, acupuncture, osteopathy and
agriculture. Since 1981 he has run a private
holistic practice in Sandefjord, Norway, for
the healing of small animals and horses, as

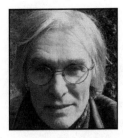

well as people. He has lectured widely, specializing in veterinary acupuncture, and has published dozens of scholarly articles. In 1984 he started to treat cancer patients, both human and animals, and this work has been the focus of much of his recent research. He is the author of *Demons and Healing* (2018), *Experiences from the Threshold and Beyond* (2019, both Temple Lodge) and several other books on complementary medicine published in various languages.

SPIRITUAL TRANSLOCATION

The Behaviour of Pathological Entities in Illness and Healing
and the Relationships between Human Beings and Animals

From Polarity to Triunity

Are Simeon Thoresen, DVM

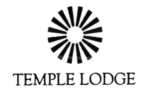

TEMPLE LODGE

Temple Lodge Publishing Ltd.
Hillside House, The Square
Forest Row, RH18 5ES

www.templelodge.com

Published in English by Temple Lodge in 2020

Originally self-published in an earlier version under the title
Translocation: An Overlooked Aspect of Medicine, Life and Spirituality and an Important Tool when Entering the Spiritual World via CreateSpace in 2019

© Are Simeon Thoresen, DVM

This new edition has been re-edited and expanded by Temple Lodge Publishing in cooperation with the author

This book is copyright under the Berne Convention. All rights reserved. Apart from any fair dealing for the purpose of private study, research, criticism or review, no part of this publication may be reproduced, stored in a retrieval system, or transmitted in any form or by any means, electronic, electrical, chemical, mechanical, optical, photocopying, recording or otherwise, without the prior written permission of the copyright owner. Inquiries should be addressed to the Publishers

The right of Are Simeon Thoresen to be identified as the author of this work has been asserted in accordance with sections 77 and 78 of the Copyright, Designs and Patents Act, 1988

A CIP catalogue record for this book is available from the British Library

ISBN 978 1 912230 45 7

Cover by Morgan Creative
Typeset by DP Photosetting, Neath, West Glamorgan
Printed and bound by 4Edge Ltd., Essex

Dedicated to All Who Seek to Heal and Understand

'After that, I asked again about pain and illness – whether much cannot be overcome through spiritual healing. [...] Frau von Moltke said that the [Christian] Scientists may well perform healing, but they drive away demons of disease and do not dissolve them, and they [the demons] can then cause further evil.'

– from a conversation between
Frau Keyserling and Frau von Moltke

Publisher's Note:
None of the medical information referred to in this book is intended as a replacement for professional advice. Any person with a condition requiring medical attention should consult a qualified medical practitioner or a suitable therapist.

Contents

Foreword

Why Did I Write This Book?

I wrote this book out of the needs I see at the present time. I see diseases being *translocated* to others—humans or animals— despite the good intentions of many therapists or doctors.

The diseases are translocated because they do not exist in energetic patterns, but as expressions of spiritual beings. Energy and energy-patterns only exist in the physical world, but in the spiritual world there are only *spiritual beings*.

This has been known in all cultures in all times and is found in all true spiritual literature. This knowledge lies at the base of all ancient religious procedures, including the 'halal' animal slaughter protocols. In ancient Israel, when millions of animals were sacrificed and their blood was washed away with water, the priests first translocated their collective sins to the animals, well aware of the phenomenon of translocation. And then, with the blood washing the sins away, i.e. translocating them further, they cleansed the sins of Israel from the Jewish tribes.[1]

When I say that I 'see' the spiritual beings being translocated, I mean through:

- clairvoyance;
- observation of how diseases develop and spread;
- observing how the treatment of one person may completely change the disease in another person or animal.

I 'see' this in connection with all forms of therapy, both in:

- orthodox allopathic medicine;
- cancer-treatment through chemo- or radiation therapy;
- homeopathy;
- acupuncture;
- herbal medicine;

- cranio-sacral therapy;
- foot-zone therapy, and a number of other therapies.

To investigate what I describe in this book, we need a certain sensitivity and/or clairvoyance; but when the connections are found, anybody can observe their validity. Two abilities are needed in order to be able to investigate these problems in the energetic-spiritual world:

- The ability to consciously cross the threshold.
- The ability to open one or more of our spiritual sense-organs.

As a therapist, doctor or veterinarian, to affect the pathological demonic entities, we also need to be able to have the following:

- The ability to act upon the spiritual phenomena that we encounter in the spiritual world, either as seekers or therapists, in order to transform what we meet.
- An understanding of the function and laws of these pathological entities and the tools to influence them. Then we can hinder the translocation and induce a real *transformation* – and by such break the endless chain of disease.

We can make a change when we have acquired a deep understanding of how to pass the threshold, how to open and use our spiritual senses and how to transform, instead of just translocate, the often-negative spiritual aspects we meet in modern society. I have written this book to try to investigate these possibilities, and to give my fellow travellers in spirit the insights, tools and ability to make such a change.

I would like to thank my publisher, Sevak Gulbekian, for his valuable editorial input in helping with my untrained English and arranging the various elements of this book. Without his backing this book would probably not have been published at all.

Introduction

The Distinction Between Energy-Patterns and Spirits

In my many courses and lectures on the subject of the various types of spiritual medicine—energetic medicine, acupuncture, homeopathy, Earth-radiation, ley lines, herbal medicine, anthroposophical medicine, general anthroposophy, and now translocation and transformation—I have experienced that one of the most difficult distinctions to make by the participants is between energy and spirit. Many of the participants in my courses are therapists, working with different kinds of energies. Energies are detectable with sophisticated instruments, and they can be 'felt' by the refined physical senses of acupuncturists working with the acupuncture points and meridians. The acupuncture points can be detected by a point-finder or by a sensitive hand or finger.

With spiritual 'energies' or 'beings' this is completely different. In the spiritual world there are no energies, although the spirit can influence the energetic world, just as the energetic world can influence the physical world. Here there are numerous levels or compartments, and these can only be reached if the observer has passed the threshold to the spirit world.[2]

The laws of the dense world are different from those of the fluid or gaseous worlds. The energetic world also has different rules, like positive or negative attraction or repulsion (a dualistic world system). This world can still be understood with the help of the Cartesian world view. 'Above' the energetic realm we meet the etheric realm, which contains the life forces. This is more spiritual that the energetic realm, and cannot be traced by physical measuring devices, but can still be observed in the growth forces of the plants and measured by the help of photons. To understand the laws in this etheric world, we need to understand quantum physics, which very few people truly understand. However, this world can be observed by several kinds of 'clear-sensing', such as those relating to sight and smell—clairvoyance and clairalience. The next realm may be called the 'astral realm', and this is totally spiritual. This can also be called the soul world, and is only observed by a still more highly-developed clairvoyance.

In this world we find several beings or spirits: ahrimanic spirits, luciferic spirits, azuric spirits, elemental spirits, nature spirits, and higher spirits like angels and archangels. In this realm, spiritual healers such as shamans work.

In this book I will not describe translocation in relation to the physical or energetic worlds, but to the *spiritual* world. That is why energetic workers like acupuncturists and medical doctors, who only work in the physical world, find this difficult to observe.

In the spiritual world everything is in motion and transition, and is in continuous development. According to Rudolf Steiner in his *Light Course*,[3] even time and space are based on movement. Also, nothing repeats itself – a specific experience can never be experienced twice. All development in the spirit is based on movement, transition, change, transformation and translocation.

In becoming clairvoyant we also have to move in the spiritual world and translocate something, or make some change in the established order of our soul properties – our spiritual make-up. Also, in treating a patient, we have to change something, make something move. We have to transform or translocate.

Quite early in my career as a veterinarian I made some astonishing observations, which were directed to finding the true cause of disease rather than focusing on the symptoms. To do this I had to learn how to develop a more sensitive spiritual observation than is usually used within ordinary veterinary or human medicine. For the most part I used (and still use) pulse diagnosis that incorporates a certain clairvoyance and general/special sensitivity.

I observed the following:

1. In treating animals, I found that the deeper, spiritual/energetic cause of the disease *almost always* was the same as the deeper cause in the owner.

2. In treating humans, I found that the deeper, spiritual/energetic cause of the symptoms *usually* was the same in the children as in the dominating parent.

3. In treating humans, I found that the deeper, spiritual/energetic cause of the symptoms *often* was the same as in the spouse, especially if the spouse was the dominating partner.

4. I found that in treating the alpha-human (the origin of the deeper cause of the disease) in a *transformative* way, a healing process was induced in the *whole* family and farm-animals.

5. I found that the use of 5-elemental thinking[4] furthers 'translocation' of the deeper cause,[5] while using systems based on 7- or 12-element thinking[6] furthers a 'transformation'. A 6-element thinking[7] furthers a 'suppression' of the symptoms. Thus:

   a. 5-element thinking is a representative for the Eastern way of thinking (Chinese, Buddhist, Hindu).

   b. 6-element thinking is a representative for the Middle-Eastern way of thinking (Islamic, Jewish).

   c. 7- or 12-element thinking is a representative for the Western way of thinking (Christian, anthroposophical).

6. When I regularly monitored the health of animals, especially horses, and they were sold to another person, the deepest cause of their symptoms changed from being like the old alpha-owner's to being like the new alpha-owner's – as soon as the animal accepted the new owner as his alpha 'master', usually after about three weeks. Also, when a young woman who was living with her dominant mother, and thus showed the same 'deficiency' as the mother, married a dominant man, she changed the deeper cause[8] within three years.

7. The described 'deeper cause' of the disease showed different symptoms, in relation to where in the body this deeper cause found its expression. A kidney weakness in the human (demonic structure related to the kidneys) remained a kidney weakness in the animal, but it expressed itself very differently, depending on where in the body 'it' (the pathological structure causing the kidney weakness) found a 'home' – found a 'hold' (see table below).

For example:

Symptoms that may arise from a poor blood circulation (the deficient process) are very variable. Symptoms differ according to the time of the year, the age and the species or breed of the animal or human patient. Poor blood circulation (in acupuncture called TH, Triple Heater) manifests differently with different species, gender and ages.

Species, gender and age	Poor blood circulation manifests as
Children	Otitis media
Young girls and boys	Eczema
Pubescent girls	Menstrual problems, painful
Pubescent boys	Acne
Older women, menopausal women	'Heat' Syndromes (internal heat after menstruation); hot flushes (vasomotor disorders)
Grown up men	Back pain
Puppies	Red skin infections around the nose
Young dogs	Furunculosis, skin infections of the paws
Trotters	Fetlock, or navicular disorders, especially on the right forelimb
Cows	Mastitis

8. I found that if there were no 'homes' or 'holding places' in the beta-human or child or animal, the transferred disease, the pathological information, the weakness or the demonic entity was not allowed to come to expression, but remained dormant (sub-clinical).

As we will see later in this book, and as it is described in several of my other books,[9] the reason for all these observations, and also the only logical explanation, is that diseases are expressions of spiritual beings—distorted (changed) elemental beings or 'demons' (pathological elemental beings). These beings are able to travel from a human being to an animal, between humans and also between animals.

In treatment the easiest way to 'heal' a person is merely to translocate the problem, i.e. the demon. It is more difficult to transform the demon. That is why several schools, especially in China, have this knowledge and try to translocate the demons into plants or semiprecious stones.[10]

When I presented these findings at the World Congress of Veterinary Acupuncture in Wrocław, Poland, in September 2019, two doctors from Taiwan stood up and said: 'We know this very well in China, but most therapists don't care about it. Some care and try to make the translocated demonic entity go into a plant or a stone, and a very few moral therapists take it upon themselves, but they get very sick and often die early.'

Most European schools of acupuncture also have this knowledge, but are not consciously aware of it, as they actually teach their students how to avoid a translocation to themselves, but do not consider that the disease can translocate to others.

With this understanding and insight, I will summarize the most important concepts that will be the foundation of all the further understandings in this book:

- All physical phenomena have a spiritual foundation, a spiritual reality.
- In the spiritual world all spiritual reality is based on spiritual entities, which means that all physical phenomena are expressions of spiritual entities.

- In the spiritual world all entities, or part of an entity, can translocate and/or transform – both the beneficial and the adversarial ones.
- When a beneficial entity or part of one translocates or transforms, our level of consciousness is changed, as well as the consciousness of the translocated/transformed entity.
- When a malignant or adversarial entity, or part of this entity, translocates or transforms in a negative way, disease is created, aggravated or translocated.
- All diseases or symptoms in humans, animals and plants are physical expressions of the presence of non-beneficial spiritual entities.
- These spiritual, non-beneficial entities might be toxic plant spirits, bacterial spirits, viral spirits, old karmic spirits or other forms of demonic spirits.
- All such pathological spirits seek a home or living place in the body – an empty or weak void to slip into.
- All adversarial spirits are of three different kinds, sometimes operating on their own, sometimes operating together, as in cancer (as will see we later). The three kinds are:
    - ahrimanic spirits
    - luciferic spirits
    - azuric spirits
- All the different symptoms in both humans and animals come from one or more of these three spiritual 'demon-families', entering through one of the twelve sense-openings and taking possession of one of twelve possible voids (the twelve main organs) in the body.
- The demons may enter via the twelve different sensory organs of the body, each belonging to one zodiacal energy stream. Twelve openings, twelve places of settling down and three types of demons – this makes 432 different possibilities, which can give rise to 1,000 symptoms in different species and different individual humans.
- All these different symptoms can be treated by addressing:
    - the void or empty space or weakness in one of the organs, thus expelling the demonic structure;

- luciferic symptoms (excessive symptoms), thus causing a translocation;
- ahrimanic symptoms (deficient symptoms), thus creating either a translocation or a transformation;
- the Middle, as we will describe later, thus causing a
transformation of the demonic entity or structure;
- the fundamental cause, the original 'demon', usually
coming from the dominant alpha-human. This original demon may be treated in all the above described
ways.
- All internal diseases in animals come from humans (they
are translocated from the alpha-human to an animal).
- In treatment or therapy, all diseases can either be *translocated* or *transformed* (not the symptoms, but the causative
'demon'). To understand the mechanism of such translocation we need to understand the following:
  - The development and spiritual construction of the
  entire cosmos.
  - The development and spiritual construction of man.
  - The development and spiritual construction of animals.
  - The reality and substance of the translocated disease.
- To be able to diagnose the diseases spiritually, we have
to enter the spiritual world through our *feeling* and also
develop some kind of 'monitoring' of these pathological
entities, as for example through the use of pulse diagnosis
or some other sort of clairvoyance.
- To be able to treat the diseases spiritually, we have to enter
the spiritual world through our *will*, and also develop some
kind of method to 'influence'.
- These pathological entities inside the patient's body, for
example through herbs, acupuncture, homeopathy or osteopathy.
- The effect of both diagnosis and treatment is highly dependent on the insights and knowledge of the therapist.
- Christ is the only transforming force.

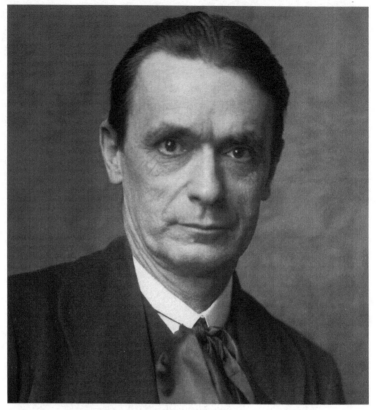

Rudolf Steiner, 1916

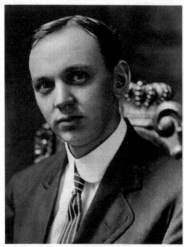

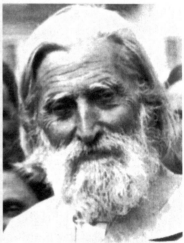

Edgar Cayce, 1911   *Peter Deunov (date unknown)*

This book is based on my own experiences, my own understanding and my own clairvoyant observations within human medicine, veterinary medicine and spirituality. It is also based on the teachings of Rudolf Steiner,[11] and to a lesser extent those of Edgar Cayce[12] and Peter Deunov.[13]

Rudolf Steiner on the concept of shared diseases

In his lectures on the *Gospel According to Luke*,[14] Rudolf Steiner discussed the importance of the concept of shared demonic pathology among all beings and its treatment with Christ Consciousness:

> At the time of Christ's appearance on the Earth there were many human beings in His environment in whom sins and transgressions—especially defects of character deriving from former bad traits—were expressing themselves in disease. The sin that is actually seated in the astral body and manifests as illness is called 'possession' in The Gospel of St Luke. It is the condition that sets in when a man attracts alien spirits into his astral body and when his better qualities fail to give him mastery over his whole nature. In human beings in whom the old state of separation between the etheric and physical bodies still persisted, the effects of evil qualities and attributes expressed themselves conspicuously at that time in forms of illness manifesting as 'possession'. The Gospel of St Luke tells how such people were healed through the mere proximity and the words of the individuality of Christ Jesus and how the evil power working in them was expelled. This is a prefiguring of conditions at the end of Earth evolution, when man's good qualities will exercise a healing influence upon all his other traits.

The above excerpt describes possession in those that suffer from the vestiges of their misdeeds, and their cure through the mere words or presence of Christ. Steiner goes on:

> When Christ speaks of 'deeper sin' — sin which reaches into the etheric body — He uses a particular expression, clearly indicating that the spiritual factor causing the illness must first be removed.

He does not immediately say to a paralyzed man: 'stand up and walk!' but concerns Himself with the cause that is penetrating as illness into the etheric body, and says: 'Thy sins are forgiven thee!' — meaning that the sin which had eaten its way right into the etheric body must first be expelled.

The above demonstrates that the cause of disease begins at the spiritual level with sin.[15]

In outer life itself, the effect made by one astral body upon another is quite obvious. You can, for example, wound a man by a word charged with hatred. Something then takes place in his astral body; he hears the word and suffers pain in his astral body. That is an example of mutual action between one astral body and another. Mutual action between one etheric body and another is far more deeply hidden; this involves delicate influences, which play from man to man but are never perceived today. The most deeply hidden of all are the influences which reach the physical body, because owing to its dense materiality it conceals the working of the spiritual almost completely.

The above paragraph explains the effects of emotions on one astral body to another, and more sinister influences that are spread from one etheric body to another that can reach to the physical. Steiner continues:

Christ Jesus shows that He is able to see into the very depths of the physical corporeality and to work into it. When it is a matter of working spiritually, man cannot be regarded as a being enclosed in his skin. It has often been said that our finger is wiser than we are ourselves. Our finger knows that the blood can flow through it only if the blood is circulating normally through the whole body; our finger knows that it would wither away if it were severed from the rest of the organism. So, too, if he would understand the conditions relating to the physical body, man must know that in respect of his physical organism he belongs to humanity as a whole; that influences are continually passing from one human being to another, and that he can in no way separate his physical health as an individual from the health of the whole of humanity.

The passage above clearly relates to the fact that we are all deeply interconnected with one another and that we translocate disease to each other. In Luke it is described thus:

> Then a man named Jairus, a synagogue leader, came and fell at Jesus' feet, pleading with him to come to his house because his only daughter, a girl of about twelve, was dying. As Jesus was on his way, the crowds almost crushed him. And a woman was there who had been subject to bleeding for twelve years, but no one could heal her. She came up behind him and touched the edge of his cloak, and immediately her bleeding stopped.[16]

Steiner comments as follows:

> How can the twelve-year-old daughter of Jairus possibly be healed, for she is at the very point of death? This can only be understood if we know that the girl's physical illness was connected with another phenomenon in another person, and that she could not be healed independently of that other phenomenon. When this child, now twelve years old, was born, a certain connection existed with another personality — a connection deeply grounded in karma. Hence, we are told that a woman who had suffered from a certain illness for twelve years, passed behind Christ and touched the border of His garment. Why is this woman mentioned? It is because she was connected karmically with Jairus' child! This twelve-year-old girl and the woman who had suffered for twelve years were deeply connected! And it is not without reason that a secret of number is indicated here: the woman with an illness suffered for twelve years approaches Jesus and is healed — and only now could He enter the house of Jairus and heal the twelve-year-old girl who was believed to be already dead.

This important section demonstrates Steiner's explanation of karma's important role among us, and how Christ can work through the higher 'I' to heal us from the ego, astral, etheric and physical body. Steiner continues:

> Your Ego, in the present stage of its development, is still weak; as yet it has little mastery. But it will gradually become master of the astral body, the etheric body and the physical body, and will transform them: the great Ideal of Christ, who reveals to mankind

what this mastery can mean! It is upon truths such as these that the Gospels are founded — truths which could be recorded only by those who did not rely upon outer documents but upon the testimony of people who were 'seers' and 'servants of the word'. Conviction of what lies behind the Gospels can be acquired only by degrees. But people will gradually grasp with such intensity and strength the nature of the truths upon which the scriptures are founded, that this understanding will have an effect upon all the members of humanity.

Rudolf Steiner states that although now our higher I, our connection to the cosmos as a singular divinity is only in its rudimentary stage, it will someday develop and flourish, at which time we will join Christ as a spiritual unity.

Chapter 1

Disease and Pathological Entities

Diseases have many different causes, such as:

- over-strengthening of the ahrimanic forces inherent in the material body,[17] due to 'ahrimanic sins';
- over- strengthening of the luciferic forces inherent in the material body, due to 'luciferic sins';
- living over 'Earth radiation', the karmic residues of others, that strengthen either our ahrimanic or luciferic structures;
- by 'wrong living', which creates a void or passage for different demons from other human beings in the past or present.

All of the translocated diseases are translocated from the 'strongest' (alpha-being) human being to a 'lesser' human or to an animal, i.e. to a being of lesser strength. This is why diseases almost never translocate from animals to humans, although this can happen. Likewise, weaker humans and children are usually the target of translocation.*

As I have indicated earlier, the ahrimanic and luciferic forces that cause disease, either by being too strong or by being received by another person, have to be transformed. If they are 'treated' directly and symptomatically, they tend to translocate. They also tend to translocate if someone 'opens' themselves to the unbalanced person, such as a spouse, children or animals. Then they will become sick from the translocated forces or entities.

We have then to understand:

- *What is translocated?*
- *How can such translocated 'things' cause disease?*

People have asked or commented on the role of karma in such translocation. Of course, those that 'attract' or 'receive' the translocated demons are already 'prepared', or karmically destined, to do so – but that does not remove the guilt from the person who intervened by expelling the demons, as they had the possibility to *transform* them.

The first time I witnessed such a 'thing' was in Bodø in 1980, when I was a veterinarian in this area of Northern Norway. A friend was visiting my wife and, when I came into the room, I *saw* a 'structure' that appeared half way out of the left side of her friend's skull, with the other half within her head. It was like a spiral, similar to a curled snake or a skein of wool. She told me that she was suffering from a painful migraine. I went towards this woman and took hold of the energetic 'structure' with my hand. I pulled the 'structure' half way out, and the woman said that the pain diminished, almost disappeared. Then I let go of the 'structure', and it slipped immediately back into the head of the woman. 'Ow', she said, 'now the pain has come back'!

Again, I grabbed hold of the 'structure' and pulled it all the way out. The migraine totally disappeared. I was very careful with what I did to the 'structure' that I held in my hand. I went to the open window, and threw the 'structure' out. It did not return.

In the following years, in fact until today, I have often asked myself:

- *What was that structure, from where had it come and where did it go after I threw it out of the window?*
- *Did it come back?*
- *Did it go to someone else?*

These questions became very important for me. The answers are essential to understanding the existence of such pathological structures (in this book referred to as 'demons'), how they are translocated and their part in disease, especially the human-animal pathological connection.

Often when I have treated diseases with homeopathy or acupuncture—which I have used much in my practice on animals and their owners—the symptoms moved around in the body. Over three to four months of repeated treatment, a migraine could move down into the hand and remain as a pain in the person's little finger for some time before it vanished into thin air. As a medically-trained person, I know that migraine is caused by a pulsating artery that affects a nerve in the head, so this moving around appeared quite strange to me – quite inexplicable.

I then had to pose the very important question to myself: *'What is it that travels from the brain into the little finger and after a while disappears?'*

Then I began to see and understand more and more what the reality behind the 'travelling structures' of diseases were. They are structures that seem to have their own life and can travel in the body from top to bottom, or vice versa. They can also jump over to another person, or to an animal. Not only *can* they do this, but jumping and travelling and changing is a fundamental property of these demons.

These structures are alive. Ordinary treatment with physiotherapy, osteopathy, acupuncture, painkillers and other allopathic medicines usually only move these structures to other places in the body (creating different symptoms than were there originally), or to other individuals, where they also create totally different symptoms, or sometimes the same symptoms.

In discussing this phenomenon with colleagues – acupuncturists, zone therapists and even Qigong therapists – I have found that they are all aware of the danger that such entities can 'jump over' to themselves, and they are very careful to prevent this from happening. To prevent this is actually a part of their education. Very few have given proper and serious consideration to the thought that such pathological entities can jump over to others—to the wife or neighbour when they come home, to the horse when they go to the stable, or to their children!

In my practice, as well in the practices of all my colleagues, I became painfully aware that we all mainly just translocate the noxious structures called 'demons' (the symptoms), and for this we receive payment!

If one reviews the literature of various alternative medical systems, there are revelations that show this translocation phenomenon was already being observed by some of the great physicians of homeopathy, such as Dr Constantine Hering,[18] the author of 'Hering's Law of Cure'.[19]

The name 'demon' calls forth disbelief in many readers. I could have described these demonic entities as 'pathological or noxious structures of either yin or yang quality with their own life', but this would not be honest.

I prefer to call them by their traditional name—demons.

- The 'pathological or noxious structure of yin quality with its own life', I will call an ahrimanic demon.
- The 'pathological or noxious structure of yang quality with its own life', I will call a luciferic demon.[20]
- The 'pathological or noxious structure of shen quality with its own life', I will call an azuric demon.

When we treat, either with materialistic methods like painkillers, antibiotics, cortisone or chemo/radiation-therapy, there is but one possible outcome from a seemingly successful treatment:

- The pathological structure is translocated either:
  - within our own body, or;
  - out of the body, searching for other victims or other bodies in which to abide.

When we treat, either with homeopathy, acupuncture or herbs, there are two possible outcomes from a seemingly successful treatment:

- The pathological structure is transformed, and:
  - the transformed structure is re-incorporated in our spiritual make-up, or;
  - the transformed structure is expelled, now as a *light* being.

- The pathological structure is translocated, either:
  - within our body, or;
  - outside our body, searching for other victims or other bodies.

If we treat the symptoms (which we may call the excess), or even if we treat the cause (which we may call the deficiency), the pathological structure may just be transposed/translocated. We think, then, that the disease is healed, but it is just hidden, symptomatically changed, moved or translocated to another being.

I have observed this occurrence for a long time, both for myself and for my colleagues. I would say that it happens in the following proportions:

- 100% of all allopathic (mainstream Western medicine) treatments.
- 90% of all alternative treatments, when the excess is addressed; that is, the area of pain or symptoms.
- 60% when the deficiency is addressed, i.e. when treated with the 5-element system.
- It rarely happens from a treatment using the 7- or 12-element system.
  - Seldom when the 90^0 method is used.
  - Sometimes when the star-method is used (see p. 53).
  - Almost never when the Middle point is addressed.[21]

In these more recent years, the most important question for me has been how to dissolve or transform the disease-causing elementals called demonic structures or demons, and not just to translocate them to others.

This described translocation gives the foundation of the observed pathological connection between all living entities.

There is a strong energetic connection between all levels of creation, and we are all connected energetically through the existence of elementals,[22] both benign beings and malign beings or so-called demons.

Three Types of Demons

In the spiritual world, on the other side of the threshold, there are many kinds of entities, just as in the physical world. Here in the physical world, we may meet innumerable types of beings – some are beneficial to us, some are indifferent and some are dangerous. In the spiritual world it is just as in the physical world, and those beings or entities that are dangerous to us we call 'adversaries'.

There are many different types of these adversaries, but to make it easier to define them we may divide them into three groups:

- The ahrimanic beings, which are adversarial entities in the etheric realm. They want us to be more materialistic and deny the spiritual world.
- The luciferic beings, which are adversarial entities in the astral realm. They want us to lose ourselves in our own subjective experiences of the spiritual world.
- The azuric beings, which are adversarial entities in both the physical and spiritual realms, attacking the physical body as well as the 'I organization'. They want us to lose our 'I', or make the 'I' egoistic and unsuitable for the spiritual world.

All diseases have their origin in the spiritual world, caused by the presence of demonic structures.

How are Demons Created?

I have come to understand that all demons are created by evil or egoistic deeds of humans, and feed on:

a. The upward-streaming forces of the deeper layers the Earth, i.e. the fifth to the ninth layers (see my book *Demons and Healing*).
b. The reflected incoming etheric forces from the surrounding cosmos.
c. The continued sinful or wrong way of thinking, feeling and will in the human host.

If the human being that created the elemental demon is dead, a grid-line in the Earth – which today we call 'Earth-radiation' – still remains as a trace or mark of the deed. During the period when the originator of the grid-line has entered the spiritual world, i.e. is dead, the grid-line remains here in the physical world. It may cause disease or discomfort in other humans or animals that happen to sleep or live where the lines are. In a later life, when the originator of the line is reincarnated, the spirit of this reincarnated human is drawn to the site where 'the line' awaits. When he or she then comes again to the area of past sin – the past misdeed – the grid-lines (demons) attach to the human, who then consciously or unconsciously remembers these past actions. It is known within criminology that the perpetrator always returns to the site of the crime.

These lines or grids contain the whole history of our lives, and are called the Akashic Chronicle.[23] Karma and the Akashic Chronicle are interwoven in this grid, and are two parts or realities of Earth radiation.

It must be understood that the whole world is full of these demons: demonic grids fed by the upward-streaming of ahrimanic forces from the depths.

They are of many kinds and appearances. Some are made by greed, others from anger, as a result of murder, violence, jealousy and from pain or sorrow.

Demons will also be created through deeds of violence towards nature.

If we cut down a tree; if we kill weeds or insects by the help of chemicals (e.g. Roundup); if we slaughter a healthy cow or horse; or if we cut down whole areas of forest with huge machines, strong disharmonic demons will be created that later can translocate both to humans and animals.

As I have already stated, demons are always involved in the development of disease that occurs in animals and in man.

Concerning diseases in humans, relating to both body and soul, the most significant demons are those we have created ourselves through our actions, thoughts and feelings. They may be called our karmic demons, or the karmic doppelgänger.

Example

I was visiting a friend of mine. He was often thrown into severe depressions, and could not work for weeks or months. He had no idea where these depressions came from. At the time I was visiting him he was in a better state. I sat at the table and he went to the kitchen to make me a coffee. As he was doing this, a huge dark shadow slowly engulfed him, and he sank into a dark mood. This dark mood that descended upon him was the cause of his repeated depressions. I tried to ask the demon from whence it came, but it would not answer. I asked the entity further how old it was, and finally it responded that it had been created by a dark action committed by my friend's grandfather. The action had to do with an act of low morality.

The next step would be to find out what this was, and then to ask for forgiveness. If these actions are properly performed, the demon will disperse and vanish, having been freed and transformed. We must not just push the demon away. It wants to be transformed.

Demons and Earth Radiation

These etheric forces from the depths of the Earth are very central to understanding the nature of demons and disease. My development in seeing and understanding Earth radiation is much the same as my path in seeing and understanding pathologic demons. I understood from early on that they belong together – that they are one and the same.

Since 1972, I have been investigating ley lines and Earth grids—so-called 'Earth radiation'—especially since 2004, when I began to *see* this matrix of energy.[24] This energy is *spiritual energy*, as no one has as yet been able to prove the existence of it with electronic instruments or other kinds of measuring devices. It can only be detected by living beings.

I am aware that there is also a huge grid of electromagnetic energy (EMR) that causes disease in living beings. This is especially noticeable in connection with emissions from high-voltage installations, 4/5G masts and cell phones. The pathological effect from EMR is actually not caused by the radiation itself, but from the adversarial forces that 'ride' the EMR. *The pathological effect from such EMR can be eliminated by using the Middle Point or the Christ-force!*

The *spiritual energy* on which the demons are feeding is an emanation from the demonic layers of the Earth itself. At the same time, it is also the expression of the demonic entities created by human misdeeds throughout all times. This 'spiritual substance' is thus both the demonic entities themselves and a kind of fuel or food for the demonic entities.

Such emanations fuel the karmic demons and cause disease, especially if one sleeps above this radiation or is connected to it.

This matrix or grid of Earth-radiation is changeable – *it is alive and has its own intent, as all spiritual beings in the spiritual world have.*

The next level of my observation was as follows: I discovered that the lines of Earth-radiation not only changed but moved several metres by themselves, especially if someone tried to alter, disperse or stop them.

Then I made the astonishing observation that they could also *be moved by my own will and intent.* I started to demonstrate this possibility to dowsers. During a dowsing congress, I moved a ley-line through the room so fast that many of the participants felt it like a soft wind that swept through the room. To me, this is proof that such 'energies' are real spiritual beings and not just 'energy'.

I carry out this moving of Earth-radiation according to the following method: first I have to 'see' the energetic lines.[25] After seeing the energy (the 'snakes') I fixate it with my willpower, just as one might call to attention a naughty child. Then, I move the 'snake' by willpower and intent to another place.[26]

In the Old Norse book *The Edda*,[27] a similar structure or phenomenon as 'Earth-radiation' and the deep up-streaming forces of the Earth is described, relating to the Norns.[28] The Old Vikings 'saw' that when a child was born, a 'web' was waiting for it. Three women were waiting to connect the child to this web, which was the karma of the new-born being. The names of the three women were past, present and future (Vilje, Ve and Verdande). The Norns also had scissors to cut the thread when the task of this life was fulfilled. This is for me an accurate description of the karmic web, the cause of its existence and how it is created. I observe this karmic web in connection with all human beings.

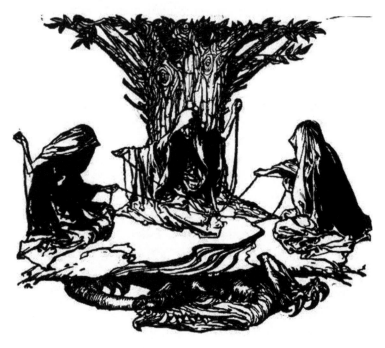

The Three Norns Weaving by Arthur Rackham

When I started to understand this, I began to see clearly the connections between Earth-radiation and humans. I saw how the actions of man created or attracted (through translocation) the snakes/demons, and how these demons created diseases and disasters for mankind.

Such demons may also create disease in people who live close by or are attached to those who carry the demons (through translocation).

It has been observed throughout time that living or sleeping above Earth-radiation may cause disease, and also that it is impossible to free yourself from these demons, unless you know how to.

This phenomenon must be described as a sort of translocation, and if we are able to correct or repent our karma, it can become transformation.

The Void

When an elemental spirit, a demon or any other benign or malign spirit enters you, influences you or actually possesses you, there must be an empty 'room' available within, i.e. some weakness or a void into which it is possible to penetrate and dwell. This is of utmost importance to know relating to:

- spiritual possession;
- use of alcohol or drugs;
- development of diseases;
- hypersensitivity; and
- exposure to electromagnetic radiation (which still contains the ahrimanic and luciferic forces that 'ride' on it).

In the beginning of man's evolution, we ourselves used this method or possibility of entering or possessing other beings, entering into the void of their spiritual construction.

As we will see in far greater detail in the following chapter, when the first group of human souls entered the Earth-sphere in Lemurian times, they entered into or actually possessed animal forms, in order to experience the pleasures of earthly existence (in Genesis they were called 'the sons or daughters of man'). But alas, they were trapped in these forms, and unable to re-enter the spiritual world.

The next group of souls entering the earthly realm was the 'rescue party' that came to help the trapped 'sons or daughters of man' back to God – incarnating in human forms which later were developed to reach the perfection of life that can house a conscious 'I'. This second group (in Genesis they were called 'the sons or daughters of *God*') came to help or rescue the first group and to free them from the material prison they had put themselves in. This second group was also trapped deeply in materialism, due to the cunning plans of the adversary, and in the end Christ himself had to come to rescue them all.

According to Rudolf Steiner, the animal forms were created as side-products of human development, but still some of the immature human souls incarnated too soon in apes and higher animals – who must be considered as our brothers and sisters, and thus need our help and salvation.

A healthy human being fills out his or her physical body to a large extent with the physical (i.e., the divine blueprint of man and also the energetic streams called by Steiner 'the invisible man within us'[29]), the etheric, astral- and 'I'-organization. But there are very few healthy humans; we are all weakened somewhat and somewhere, depending on our individual lives, individual karma and individual beliefs.

Just after we are born, a 'demonic being' takes possession of our physical body, using it to stay with us for our whole life. Just before death, this being takes its leave. This ahrimanic being is called our 'doppelgänger', which is described in Rudolf Steiner's lecture of 16 November 1917.[30]

This entity is just one of the many entities that may possess us throughout our lives and make use of our body, our etheric body, our astral body or 'I'-organization.

It is important to understand that how we eat, how we think or act, as well as our moral behaviour, influence our lives and create certain weaknesses in our spiritual/physical make-up. Such weaknesses create portals through which alien spirits or spiritual influences may enter.

If, for example, we have no consciousness about our food and eat fast food every day – such as is found, say, at McDonalds – then, after a few weeks or months, our liver will become so weakened in its etheric make-up that it will be open to an alien invasion or to the creation of adversarial entities. An ahrimanic spirit can develop from our own etheric forces, or an existing ahrimanic demon can enter. This creates a 'deficient' disease, as symptoms in such a case always show a lessening of activity. This ahrimanic, elemental demonic entity invites or creates a luciferic demon, and this demon reveals symptoms that are considerably clearer than those caused by the ahrimanic one, and this is called an 'excessive' disease. Therefore, most diseases are a cooperation between ahrimanic and luciferic demons – the luciferic dwelling cranial (towards the head) and the ahrimanic dwelling distal (towards the feet). Between these two we find the Middle Point, or the area I call the 'Christ Point'. If we strengthen this area, the two adversarial forces will be transformed and weakened.

Other causes for opening up an invasion of adversarial forces may be the use of alcohol and drugs. If, for example, there is too big an opening in the defensive power of the body due to a weakening of one's etheric or astral strength, certain portals may be created, and through such portals alien entities or influences may enter. The result is often seen as hypersensitivity and allergies. The hypersensitivity of electromagnetic radiation (EMR) is a very striking example.

There are, to my knowledge, four ways in principle to help or treat such an influx of entities or unwanted spirituality, due to having too wide an opening of portals or a weakening of the protective force of the etheric or astral sheaths:

1. To *translocate* the spirits (as in exorcism).
2. To make room for the Christ-force in the Middle, in order to *transform* the unwanted luciferic or ahrimanic spirits.
3. To *close the 'door'* that allows the spirits in.
4. To *fill the void*, by changing one's detrimental way of living.

The 'Planned' Void of the Brain and the Heart

According to Rudolf Steiner, part of the divine plan to rescue humanity from the curse of materialism was put in motion in 1721, when preparations for the spiritualization of man began. The first move was slowly to part the etheric body from the head, so that it would be possible to develop connections to the spiritual world, and also to develop clairvoyance.

Later, in the 1900s, the etheric body started to separate from the heart, so that spiritual activity had the possibility to develop in the heart region.

This means that all the forces, of both the head and the heart, concerning the etheric body, astral body and 'I' are free from the material body and as such are free to work in the spiritual realm. If this work is not done, if the void is not filled out with one's own spirituality, then luciferic, ahrimanic and/or azuric forces may slip in and take possession of our humanity, and waves of disease may result.

Chapter 2

Understanding Translocation Through Knowledge of the Development of Man and Animal

In this chapter, I will describe the background to the mechanism of translocation through understanding the development of both man and animal, as well as the development of Earth and cosmos.

The Development of The Animals

The beginning of the creation of the higher animals started on Old Moon,[31] an earlier incarnation of our Earth, with the development of what has been called 'animal-man'-creatures. When present day Earth developed, the less developed part of the animal-man population did not wait for proper human forms to develop, and incarnated in animal forms. They were thus trapped in these bodies.

The more developed souls waited until these bodily forms were mature enough to receive a being that could incarnate an 'I'-consciousness. These souls became people – the human kingdom. The human archetype waited for a much longer time in the spiritual world until it found a body mature enough to incarnate in. The less-developed humans entered those immature forms which could not support an 'I'-being. These beings then had to leave their spiritual 'I' in the spiritual world, and this 'I'-consciousness stayed in the spiritual world, as the 'I' of the group soul of that particular animal species.

In 1904, Rudolf Steiner said:

> ... simultaneously with its first incarnation in the beginning of the Lemurian age, the untarnished human spirit ... sought its primal physical incarnation. The physical development of the Earth with

its animal-like creatures had not evolved so far at that time that it could incarnate the human spirit, the human 'I'. But a part of it, a certain group of animal-like beings had evolved so far that the seed of the human spirit could descend into it to give form to the human body.[32]

Edgar Cayce has a quite special story of the Beginning, in which the first humans somewhat prematurely incarnated into physical bodies. According to Cayce, the first men came down to Earth too early, because they were tempted by experiences of the flesh, especially sexual experiences. They then became trapped in the material realm, although that was something they did not intend. They had wanted to remain for just a short while. As mentioned earlier, in the Bible they were then called the sons and daughters of man (Genesis 6, 1-6).[33]

Consequently, a rescue team was sent down by command of God the Creator, to lead the fallen humans (those that had fallen into animal forms) back to God again – and so we have the present situation today, where the animal kingdom must be rescued by the human kingdom.

A solution to enable liberation of the souls entangled in matter was created by the spiritual world. First a physical form became available as a vehicle for the 'rescue-party' souls descending to Earth. Thus, a way was created for these souls to enter the Earth and experience it as part of their evolutionary/reincarnation cycle. Of the physical forms already existing on Earth, the most appropriate to fulfil the required bodily form was a species of anthropoid ape-man. Souls descended upon these apes – hovering above and around them rather than inhabiting them, and influenced them to move towards a different goal to the simple one they had been pursuing. These creatures then left their tree habitations, built fires, made tools, lived in communities and began to communicate with one another. Eventually, they lost their animal appearance, shed bodily hair, and took on refinements of manner and habit.

The evolution of the human body occurred partly through the souls' influence on the endocrine glands, until the ape-man was a three-dimensional objectification of the soul hovering above it.

In this manner the soul fully descended into the physical body, giving the Earth a new inhabitant: 'Homo sapiens'. Homo sapiens appeared in five different places on Earth at the same time, creating the five broad 'races' that exist today. This evolved human being is what the Bible refers to as 'Adam'.

When souls incarnated into physical form, they brought divine consciousness (i.e., the spirit) with them. Cayce referred to this divine consciousness as the 'Christ Consciousness', 'Buddhahood' or the 'super consciousness'. Christ Consciousness has little to do with the personality known as Jesus. It means a person has attained a complete human-divine unity. This human-divine unity has been attained by many people thus far – and one such person was Jesus, according to Cayce. According to Rudolf Steiner, many personalities throughout history may have experienced a 'Christ consciousness', but only in Jesus of Nazareth did the entire being of the 'Second Logos of the Sun-Trinity' – the *Son*, the Christ-being himself – incarnate.

The problem for the soul entangled in flesh was to overcome the attractions of the Earth to the extent that the soul would be as free within the body as out of it. Only when the body was no longer a hindrance to the free expression of the soul could the Earth cycle be completed. This is the condition of having a perfect unity of the human with the divine. In a more focused perspective, this was the evolutionary drama of free will and creation. In a still more focused perspective, each atom of the physical body is a world unto itself, where a drama of free will and creation is occurring. The soul brings life into each atom, and each atom is a physical reflection of the soul's pattern.

With the advent of consciousness, humans became aware that the sexual act meant more to them than it did to the animal world. Sexual activity is the 'door' through which new souls enter the Earth, a door which is unnecessary in other heavenly planetary/realms. Sexual activity is thus the only means which trapped souls have of being liberated from their predicament – through the cycle of birth, death and rebirth.

I will here refer further to a 1936 reading by Edgar Cayce (no. 1183-1). This mentioned 'giants' in Lemuria. According to

Cayce, Lemuria, or Mu, was a land based in the South Pacific that was all but destroyed by 50,000 BC. Cayce related that there were many changes happening to the physical surface of the Earth at that time (upheavals and natural disasters) and that the 'sons and daughters of men' were interacting with 'the sons of the daughters of God'. According to the reading, many thought forms were projecting themselves into physical form on Earth and 'monsters' were present. Many of these were large, dangerous animals that roamed in herds causing destruction. Most Cayce scholars believe he was referring to mastodons, mammoths and mega-fauna such as sabre tooth tigers and giant sloths. But various of his readings refer to 'things'—animal monstrosities. In some readings, Cayce related that various 'things' were created, by what appears to be some form of genetic manipulation. The 1936 reading tells us that this was the time period related to in the biblical quote: 'In those days there were giants on the Earth.' The use of the terms 'sons and daughters of men' and 'sons and daughters of God' are apparently unique to Cayce, but he described the meaning of these terms in various places.

As we have seen, human life resulted from thought forms (souls) that projected themselves into physical form. But by so doing, the energy-based soul became trapped in physical matter. Cayce's term 'sons and daughters of men' refers to 'souls who had become so physical, so terrestrial as to have lost their awareness.'[34]

In losing this awareness of their true spiritual nature, the souls were destined to reincarnate into physical form until they regained awareness of their nature and origin. The 'sons and daughters of men' had evolved over many lifetimes and became physically smaller in size. But during this early time period, somewhere around 210,000 BC, more thought forms projected into physical form and they initially retained some of the knowledge of their true nature. These were called the 'sons and daughters of God' because they still had a connection to their source and remained somewhat god-like. Trapped within their encasement in physical form, the 'daughters of men' began to

interbreed with the newly arriving 'sons of God', 'creating creatures that were half god-like in their size and power and half
human'. These are referred to in the Bible as the Nephilim. Inca
legends tell of a time when bands of these gigantic, half-breed
offspring came to the shores of their land, causing havoc until
natural forces arose and rid the land of them. Many Native
American legends also tell of the arrival of giants that were can-
nibals and who eventually became rulers.

We see from this that both animals and man originate from
the same souls, the only difference being that some souls were
too eager to descend into the physical and material world. They
were trapped in animal forms and became the higher animals.
They are our brothers and sisters, and it is our duty to help them
to one day become human. We must and should treat them with
love and respect. The animals are our lost siblings and they are
connected to our future, whether we like it or not.

Every species has its own 'I' that is functioning in its group
soul in the spiritual world. Each human being has its own 'I'
whilst every animal species has its common 'I' in the higher spiritual world. Each human being has its own astral body, whilst
the animal species have their specific 'group soul' in the upper
part of the Earth's atmosphere.

Every individual animal has an astral body that is a concentrated aspect of the group soul, in which each individual animal
soul participates. The repertoire of emotions that are available to
each animal comes from the group soul, and the experiences of
each individual animal return to the group soul.

More About the Group Soul in Animals

In 1924 Rudolf Steiner wrote:

> What is it that we call instinct in the animals? We know that the
> animals have a Group soul. The animal, such as it is, is not a
> self-contained being. The Group soul is standing there behind it.
> Now, to what world does the Group soul belong? We must first

answer this question: Where do we find the Group souls of the animals? They are certainly not to be found here in the physical world of sense. Here we have only the single individual animals. We do not find the Group souls of the animals until, by initiation or in the ordinary course of human evolution between death and a new birth, we come into that altogether different world which man passes through between his successive earthly lives. There indeed we find, among the beings with whom we are then together, including above all those of whom I have been speaking to you, those with whom we elaborate our karma — there we find the Group souls of the animals. And the animals that are here on the Earth, when they act instinctively, they act out of the full consciousness of the Group souls. You may conceive it thus, my dear friends. [Dr Steiner here made a drawing on the blackboard.] Here we have the realm in which we live between death and a new birth; and out of it there work the forces which proceed from the Group souls of the animals. And here upon this Earth we have the single animals which act and move about, guided as it were by threads which pass to the Group souls — the beings whom we ourselves discover in the realm between death and a new birth. Such in truth is instinct. It is obvious that a materialistic world-conception cannot explain instinct, for instinct is: to act out of that sphere of being which you will find described as Spirit-land in my *Theosophy* for example, and in my *Occult Science*. For man however it is different. Man too has instinct, but when he acts through his instinct, he is not acting out of yonder Spirit-realm, but out of his own former lives on Earth. He is acting across time, out of his former earthly lives, out of a whole number of former lives on Earth. As the spiritual realm works upon the animals, causing them to act instinctively, so do the former incarnations of man work on his later incarnations in such a way that he instinctively lives out his karma. But this is a spiritual instinct — an instinct that works within the Ego. It is just by understanding this that we shall come to understand the absolute consistency of this instinctive working with human freedom. For the freedom of man proceeds from the very realm out of which the animals act instinctively, namely the realm of the spirit.[35]

The beginning of an individual 'I' in animals

If the group soul has opened up to human beings, either individually (which is seldom) or as a group (more usual), the species is called 'tame', or domesticated. Being 'domesticated' implies that the group soul has opened itself to the human 'I'. This opening up affects all the individuals in a species, with the exception of those members of the species that have been met with too much violence from human interaction, thus closing their 'individual openings'.

This opening of the animal group soul to the human being, to the human 'I', also means that part of, or rather a 'mirror-image', of the human 'I' is projected into the specific animal. It is as if the group soul has opened to a general influx of human soul- and 'I'-properties. This I have witnessed myself.

Example

Between the years 2005-2010 I had a horse named 'Balder'. He was a gelding of North-Swedish heritage, a firm and typically cold-blooded horse. I was closely attached to him and loved him dearly. It felt as though we could read each other's thoughts. After a long and chronic disease, I had to shoot him at the farm where we both had lived for some years. At the spot where he was shot, I could see both him (his spiritual entity) and follow his 'path' for several days. For the first two days he was somewhat angry with me for having taken his life. Then he went into his own 'purgatorio', where he fought with etheric wolves for two days. This was his deep-rooted fear – actually the fear of all horses – and they experience this vividly after death. Then a most interesting thing happened. A mare of Hanoverian breed happened to pass by. This mare also lived on our farm, and she was inseminated just a few days earlier with sperm from one of Germany's best Hanoverian stallions. When the mare passed by, the whole etheric/astral soul of Balder dissolved in a sort of mist, and this mist streamed or flowed into the stomach of the mare.

Nine months went by, and the foal was born to the Hanoverian mare. My ex-wife, who was very skilled in horse-breeding and a connoisseur of horse races, was shocked. The foal was like a 50/50 per cent mix of cold-blood and Hanoverian.

My conclusion of this happening was that, due to the love between Balder and myself, which must have involved some kind of individual soul pattern, he was able to withstand the call of the group soul and reincarnate in a somewhat different 'race', just to continue to be close to me.

We see here how the close relationship and love between humans and animals will and can lay the foundation of the development of both an individual soul (separated from the group) and an individual 'I'-consciousness, that can even reincarnate.

Many dog owners and their families have also observed how increasingly dogs take over their master's individuality. This phenomenon has to be discussed at more length, as it differs somewhat from the teachings of Rudolf Steiner (as far as I know). Rudolf Steiner describes a 'normal' change in animals that have a certain 'I'-consciousness, or individualized group soul, after death, as follows:

> Just as this describes what we begin to feel with regard to these unsuspected beings, so it is where the souls of the plants are concerned. The plant egos dwell in a higher world than the animal egos. The separate group egos of the plants live on what we call the devachanic plane. We can even state the place where they actually are — in the very centre of the Earth – whereas the animal group souls circle round the Earth, like trade winds. All these plant egos at the centre point of the Earth are mutually interpenetrating beings, for in the spiritual world a law of penetrability prevails and all beings pass through one another. We see the animal group souls moving over the Earth like trade winds, and how in their wisdom they carry out what appears to be done by the animals.[36]

The translocation from humans to animals

We will now try to imagine the animal group soul and also the animal group- 'I', and compare it to the human soul and 'I', and how these interact with each other when love arises between an animal and a human being.

There have been a multitude of observations in how different animal species can communicate, talk, remember and reason. This is seen especially in the great apes, but also in elephants, whales and dolphins, and with birds like ravens and crows. Many of these animals also have the ability to recognize themselves in a mirror. All humans who have owned and loved a dog, a cat or a horse know that they too have their own individuality. Many different observations point to the fact that animals can have a certain 'I'-function. However, other observations would suggest that they don't.

All of these controversies and differing opinions and observations can be solved by accepting the possibility of translocation. Human diseases can enter animals through the multiplying 'demon' of the disease. This also applies to translocated parts, or reflections of these parts, as well as smaller copies of the human 'I'-function through the human-animal connection, especially furthered by love between a human and an animal.

When the animal group soul becomes 'tamed', it opens up to the human soul, but also to the human 'I'. The animal species as a whole opens up to the dominion of humans, and accepts the 'taming process'. This brings these creatures the possibility of receiving all human diseases as well as bringing into being the beginning of the individual soul and the individual 'I'-consciousness.

We must again remember what Edgar Cayce described, i.e. that several of the higher animals are inhabited by human souls – or at least human souls that 'should' have been human, but due to their eagerness and impatience became trapped in animal bodies. It is possible for shamans to incarnate in these 'human-animal' bodies, as the bodies of these animals are 'familiar' with a human-like soul. If we examine the stories of indigenous people the world over, they are capable of incarnating in large birds, horses and wolves, although I personally have never heard of shamanic incarnations in dolphins or whales. The only time I myself have experienced incarnation in an animal was in a bird. It was actually quite pleasant, apart from all the troubles I had with managing the big beak, which was always in the way![37]

The animals are thus highly sentient beings, having a common group soul, as well as a 'group-I' and a gradually emerging, individual sentient soul along with an emerging 'I'-consciousness, that is linked with and dependent on the human soul- and 'I'-consciousness.

Scientists of today are accepting more and more that animals have highly developed feelings, possibly even higher than humans, and that they may indeed have entirely different feelings than we do.

This is an extremely important part of animal behaviour and disease. The owner and the veterinarian often overlook or at least underestimate the sentient ability of animals.

There is also evidence that some animals, especially dogs and cats, dream. Usually we admit that animals have feelings like fear and aggression, but many researchers believe that animals have a whole range of feelings as humans do, and maybe even more.

According to Rudolf Steiner animals experience *more* pain than humans. He stated:

> So we understand 'pain' in the astral body by conceiving it as the expression of weakness of the etheric body in relation to the physical body. An etheric body that is in harmony with its physical body works back upon the astral body in such a way that the feeling of well-being is an inner experience of health. On the other hand, an etheric body that is at odds with its physical body works back upon the astral body in such a way that pain and discomfort are bound to arise in it. Now we shall be able to realize that, because in the higher animals — it will be better to speak of the lower animals in the next lecture — the life of soul is so intimately bound up with the bodily nature, this soul experience will be much more deeply felt — as will also be the case in a disordered body — than it can be in a disordered human body.

> Because the soul life of man is emancipated from the inner, bodily experience, pain that is merely due to bodily circumstances is far less torturing, it gnaws much less deeply into the soul than in the higher animals. We can also observe that bodily pain in children is a much keener psychic pain than in later life, because in the measure in which the adult human being becomes independent of his bodily organization, he finds in the qualities which arise immediately out of his soul, the means to struggle against bodily pain; whereas the higher animal, being so closely bound up with its bodily nature, feels pain with infinitely greater intensity than man. Those who maintain that human pain can be more intense than pain felt by the animals, are talking without foundation. Pain in the animal is far, far more deep-seated than purely bodily pain in man can ever be.[38]

These include feelings like sorrow, joy, depression, elation, grief, compassion, melancholy, longing, etc. The animals may even have feelings that we do not understand or cannot imagine.

I have often observed how the emotions of the owner or stable hand influence the animals through the whole day. Many farmers report that the frequency of mastitis increases when they have weekend-help in the barn. It can be very stressful for cows to be milked by an unknown and insensitive person. The stress reaction can precipitate immunosuppression, which can allow mastitis to arise.

I have noted that a change of staff or riders is often associated with decreased performance in thoroughbred horses. This is especially marked when former staff or riders had close and good relationships with the horses, and maybe even worked overtime to make life easier for them. I have noted a long-lasting decrease in racing ability, and more infections and injuries, when a regular member of staff is replaced with someone that is much tougher or more heavy-handed.

To demonstrate the advanced sensitivity of these animals, here are two examples from my practice:

I have also noticed that noise from fans, bad smell from manure, humidity due to bad ventilation, irregular feeding and careless husbandry, highly influence meat or milk quality.

- A Norwegian horse was to be sold in Germany. At home it showed no lameness and was a very stable and friendly horse. But as soon as it arrived in Germany it became lame, got bruises, wounds and other serious problems. It was not sold. By chance I was in the area and had the opportunity to treat the horse. In investigating the animal with the help of pulse diagnosis, I found the energy in the HT meridian to be almost zero. The horse showed severe signs of sorrow, knowing it was to be sold. I treated the HT meridian, and the horse changed radically. All the problems vanished like dew to the sun. As the owner realized this connection, she immediately took the horse home again to Norway.
- Another horse was to be sold that had been free of problems for a long time, but on examination in Oslo it showed severe lameness in several legs. It was sent to my clinic where via pulse diagnosis I found a severe Qi deficiency in the HT meridian which led to a decreased blood circulation in the front legs. The horse had mourned being sold, and developed what we in humans call a bruised and broken heart. The horse was treated, and all the problems disappeared quickly.

In more relaxed and easy-going days, the old farmers in the west of Ireland had a saying: 'Look after your animals and they will look after you'. Compassion towards animals involves treating them as individuals, treating them with respect, dignity, patience, gentleness and kindness. It also involves close physical contact (massaging, scratching and rubbing the animals), talking and singing to them, and *playing with them*. Today, these aspects of animal care are not taken as seriously as they should be. The reasons for this are multiple. One reason is that modern labour is scarce and expensive. One worker must handle many more animals today than was the case in the past. Therefore, animal handlers do not have the time to get to know the individual natures, likes and dislikes of their animals. Even if they do know, they cannot, or will not, take the time to cater for individual needs or preferences in their animals.

Another important factor is that quantity rather than quality is the measure of animal productivity today. This is not so obvious in pork meat (even though many studies show the relationship between stress and meat quality) as in the objectively recorded race times in horses. Race times certainly become longer in stressed animals.

The Functional Mechanisms of Translocation

Now, after understanding something of the background development of man and animal, and how animals live, die and connect to human beings, it will be easier to understand the mechanism of translocation.

One interesting aspect of translocation is that the pathological entity – demon, spectre or phantom – almost always goes from the stronger entity to the weaker; and when it goes to this weaker entity, there must be a place for it to lodge – a void in which it can find its space, its house.

In an animal that is tamed, one that has opened its 'group soul' to mankind, either to humans in general or to a specific human, then the 'I' of the human being is always stronger than the 'part-group soul' that the animal possesses. When the animal undergoes some kind of stress or receives insufficient food, it then provides a void into which a part of the demon based in the human being can enter. The 'human demon' splits off a clone, and this clone then enters the animal and becomes an 'animal demon'.

In this way, the animal also brings the 'demon-clone' in contact with the whole group soul – and thus one single human may 'infect' a whole group of animals.

Example 1

Once I was called by a sheep farmer who lived in the upper part of Gudbrandsdalen in Norway. All of his eighty sheep had got the same problem, a definite issue with the oestrus or reproductive cycle. This occurred immediately after he had hired a new shepherdess who had come up from Oslo. He called me to ask for advice concerning his sick sheep. I immediately felt that this disease was not due to some herb containing oestrogenic; rather, it was due to translocation from a human. I asked to talk with the shepherdess, and became convinced that her menstrual and hormonal problems were the cause. I asked her to return to Oslo, and as soon as she did this the problem disappeared.

Nothing else was changed.

Example 2

I had been asked to treat a young woman with cystitis – bladder infection. She was 30 years-of-age, and had suffered from chronic cystitis for 25 years. She came together with her mother, a very special woman, 50 years-of-age. Through pulse-diagnosis I found the deficiency (treated after the 5-element thinking – a thinking which I now know furthers translocation instead of transformation), and treated her bladder. All the time, whilst I was with the 25-year-old woman, the mother was speaking about herself – how she also had been suffering from chronic cystitis for decades. It was 'me, me, me and me'! A few days later, I was called by the mother saying that her daughter was not better, but that *she* was totally cured. I was astonished, asked her daughter to come back without her, and after treating the daughter alone, she also was cured.

Example 3

A man from Oslo brought me two small dogs that had chronic pruritus (scratching) that nobody had been able to cure, not 'even' at the veterinary college. I pulsed both dogs, and found that each had a heart deficiency. I then turned to the owner and pulsed him, and found that he also had a heart deficiency. On asking him how long the two dogs had been suffering from eczema, he replied two years. I asked who had left him and caused him heartbreak about two years ago, upon which he almost burst into tears, telling me that the love of his life had left him just a month before both dogs began suffering from eczema. I then treated the owner's heart meridian, also asking him to deal with his sorrow and talk with the lost love. After two weeks, both dogs were ninety per cent better.

Example 4

For two years a German dressage horse had a severe problem in turning right. Many veterinarians, osteopaths, acupuncturists and chiropractors had tried to treat the horse, but without success. The horse did not get better. I asked the rider if I could examine her (the rider herself), and found a stuck vertebra (C4) in her neck. I manipulated this and asked her to test the horse again. She protested, as I hadn't even touched the horse, but after my insistence, she did try the horse. She put the saddle on and rode out into the riding school. Ten minutes later she came back. The horse was one hundred per cent cured.

Example 5

There is an epidemic of mammary cancer in dogs today. Likewise, there is a steadily growing number of women that get breast cancer. This is for me, and should be for many, a very obvious example of translocation.

Of course, all the examples referred to here can be explained in other ways, but if you really *see* demonic translocation, other explanations seem silly and simply uninteresting.

The Spatial Mechanism of Human-Animal Translocation

One may consider the 'tame' animals as having allowed the human spirit and soul—yes, actually the whole human spiritual makeup—to enter or communicate with both their individual souls and their group soul. When a whole species (such as the cow) has opened its group soul to the influence of humans, all individual cows will submit to human will, thoughts and feelings. The individual animal reflects this opening, and lets the specific owner or care-giver influence it. This is an opening in the group soul – in the collective group soul – and as such all animals of the species will accept the dominion of humans. This mechanism was demonstrated by the shepherdess and her flock of sheep in Gudbrandsdalen in Norway, referred to earlier. The influence or passage-way goes from the human 'I'-consciousness to the animal 'group soul'. Such a passage always goes from above to below, from the 'I' to the astral body, from the astral to the etheric, and from the etheric to the physical.

In humans, the diseases or moods in a grown-up's astral body will influence children's etheric bodies. This is very important to know for parents and teachers.

In animals, their group soul will always be influenced by the 'I' of humans. That is why humans seldom get influenced by animals. It is of course possible that the pathology of the group soul or the astral body of the animal can slip into the etheric body of a human being, causing the human to become immediately sick (zoonoses is the technical term). I saw this once at a seminar in Worpswede (Germany), where I treated a horse from the Middle Point with Christ Consciousness. After the treatment, 'something' came out of the horse, and this 'something' swirled around inside the circle of onbserving students. They really should not have been standing in a circle, as this captured the 'something' (see for example in the beginning of Goethe's *Faust*, when Mephistopheles is ensnared within a circle drawn on the floor by Faustus). Then it (the 'something') disappeared into thin air. One of the students happened to attract a part of the 'something' that was released. Returning home after the seminar, she immediately became sick. Thanks to her therapist, who was able to quickly diagnose this 'partial pathological structure' and release it, she recovered without serious damage. (How that was done, I do not know – it was probably translocated elsewhere.) The 'something' was stuck in her heart, where it tried to make its new home.

On the Group Souls of Animals

In one of his esoteric lessons (Dornach, 14 March 1924) Rudolf Steiner described how as human beings we are not contained within our skin. Rather, to spiritual consciousness the human being is as great as the universe. His thoughts are as wide as light, his feelings are as wide as warmth, and his will is as wide as air.

Thus we see that man fills up the whole cosmos, especially our solar system. Animals also do this, and the animal soul can as such be found throughout the atmosphere (see illustration below).

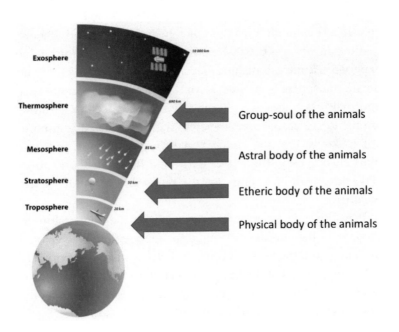

If we consider the animal soul and group soul as related to the Earth and its atmosphere, we find that the group soul is situated in the 'thermosphere' of the Earth, some 800–1,000 kilometres above the surface of the Earth (where of course the physical bodies of the animals dwell). It is at this height that the human pathological entities or demons enter the animal. This might appear to be a little strange, but the following story will perhaps make this seem more probable.

While working in Northern Norway, I had some communication with the Sami people. They have a huge knowledge about the aurora borealis, also called the northern lights. They believe – actually they *know* – that the aurora can enter your body and make you crazy, and all children are warned to be cautious. I was also told that if you had a certain feeling for animals, you could 'direct' the aurora at your wish. You just had to attract its awareness – its astral awareness – and then it would follow your wishes or directions. One night, in the darkness of the North, I was the final passenger on a boat trip home after a visit to treat a sick cow. I was in the company of a Sami man, who showed me the secret techniques of directing the aurora.

It was unbelievable! I made the aurora go where I wanted, to behave as I wanted. It was completely at my command. I knew that the aurora was 800,000 metres up in the air, and found the experience quite astonishing. This indicates that the activity in the thermosphere is in direct contact with our 'I'-consciousness, and that this consciousness can have full connection with the animal forces of that area: the animal group souls. It is important to know that the connection between humans and animals encompasses the whole Earth and its atmosphere, up to 100 kilometres, including also the possibility to influence the weather.[39]

It is also very interesting to be aware of the temperature in the area of the atmosphere where the intervention between the human 'I' and the animal group souls takes place. We normally believe or think that the higher we get, the colder it gets. This is not so. From the surface of the Earth it gets colder and colder the higher we go, but at some point it starts to get warmer.

At about 20 km above the Earth, at the ending of the tropo-sphere, it is very cold, around -60 degrees celsius. When we go further up, we reach the ozone layer in the stratosphere, about 50,000 metres up, and there the temperature is around 0.0 degrees. Then, when reaching a height of about 80,000 metres, at the beginning of the thermosphere, it sinks to -40 again. Reach-ing the middle of the thermosphere, the temperature may reach +1,500 degrees celsius – very warm indeed! In this temperature the northern lights, the aurora borealis, play out, and here the full interconnection between humans and animals takes place. That is why the human 'I' can fully and totally interfere and dominate the fluctuations of the aurora.

A further thought: Could our present cruel treatment of animals have anything to do with the climate crisis?

The Importance of Extinct Species in Translocation

We are now in the beginning—actually the middle—of the sixth great extinction of earthly species. This extinction is increasingly referred to as 'the Anthropocene Extinction', because of our actions and greed, the human being is the main cause. Due to human activity, animals are losing their habitats and foundation for life at a rapid pace. We human beings over-fish, over-exploit, pollute, deforest, mine, farm, hunt and alter the climate, so that, according to Harvard biologist E. O. Wilson, half of the Earth's species will be extinct by 2100. Other biologists estimate that around forty per cent of all species will be extinct by 2050.

How will that influence the human being and the health of the rest of the surviving animal species?

This is a very interesting question: Where do the group souls and the 'group-I's of extinct species go? When there are no lon-ger bodies in which the spiritual structures of the extinct species can incarnate, where do they go and what do they do?

As we know from the spiritual development of the cosmos, man and the animals, all existing animal species originate from the evolution of man. After death, on its way from the etheric world to the spiritual world, the human soul meets the group souls of all species in the astral world. In this astral world, the dead human entity will meet all the passions, anger and emotions expressed by animals in the animal world. If the physical mirror of some of these group souls have become extinct, then the group soul, with its strong emotions, will seek its realization in the physical world, and in this sphere will penetrate into existing species – even into the human being.

As already described, the animal etheric, astral and mirrored 'I'-function have a connection in the thermosphere to the human being, as well as to other species. This is the foundation of translocation, of our dominion over the animal world – especially the domesticated animals, but also to some extent over the non-domesticated ones too.

Chapter 3

From Translocation to Transformation

In this chapter we will see how all disease-creating demons (ahrimanic), spectres (luciferic) or phantoms (azuric) can either be translocated or transformed, and that the strongest transforming force is love. We will uncover the horrific, mind-shattering realization experienced by animal owners and veterinary therapists when they come to understand the reality that pathological entities (called demons, spectres or phantoms) can or will be translocated to other beings through the treatment of a 5-element based energetic method. These methods include conventional (or Western) medicine as well as several other healing methods that are referred to as 'natural'.

Translocation vs Transformation

As we referred to in the Introduction, there are two fundamental methods of healing:

- treating the excess, the symptoms;
- treating the deficiency, the root cause of the disease.

The first method, used widely in allopathic (Western) medicine, treats the symptoms directly. For example, one reduces a fever by giving anti-inflammatories. However, the same effect is had by using cooling herbs, or heat-dispelling acupuncture points. I have termed this method of translocation as 'treating the excess'.

Alternatively, the healer can attempt to treat at a deeper level, more commonly used in alternative medicine, by stimulating the vital force. That is, to treat the underlying fundamental weakness that created the symptoms in the first place. I have termed this as 'treating the deficiency'. Earlier in my career as a healer, I was under the assumption that the latter was the superior and more effective curative method. I now realize that both techniques are sub-optimal. This is because with both modalities the pathological entity is simply transposed to another host. However, the treatment of the excess translocates ninety per cent of diseases, whereas the treatment of the deficiency translocates only forty per cent of diseases. It has only been in the last few years of my practice that I have come to this realization, which showed itself through my treatment of cancer, as described in detail later in this chapter. When my cancer treatments stopped working after thirty years of positive results (eighty per cent total healing and remission of the cancer), I had to question the deeper foundations of this treatment. I then knew that I had to find a method that could truly annihilate the disease – to truly transform it and turn it into something good, something beneficial. This involves *activating the transformative process – which is neither the excess nor the deficiency, but something literally in-between – through love (or the Christ-force).*

- The first imperative is to localize the 'alpha-person' – the originator – of the disease, and to treat that person.
- The second imperative is to treat the original demon or demonic structure in a transformative way, not one that simply translocates it.

How to practice these imperatives will be explained below.

Introduction to My Cancer Therapy

Three decades ago, when I began adopting the modalities of homeopathy and acupuncture, I enjoyed a substantial degree of success in helping my patients. I continued to increase the efficacy of these treatments by adding the innovative use of both acupuncture 'ting-points'[40] to treat equine pathology (1982) and the control cycle of 5-element acupuncture in the treatment of cancer in both humans and animals (1984).

However, as we have seen, later I came to the discovery that my treatments actually often enforced a translocation of the disease to other persons and animals.[41] From my experience, almost all diseases in animals are translocated from their own-ers in a 'natural' way, but traditional 'alternative' treatments actually enforce this.* I gradually realized, through both careful observation of pathological symptoms in whole families and also from direct spiritual sight, that the pathological entities that were causing the illness were not transformed, and that my ear-lier 'success' did not actually result in a true cure. In fact, I was merely exteriorizing these entities, allowing their transmission to another host. Furthermore, I concluded that these adversaries were quite resistant to what I call 'transformation'.[42]

The process of transformation can be likened to disarming these noxious stimuli, rendering them free of malicious intent and rehabilitating them with qualities that will actually help – rather than hinder – mankind.

Observing my cancer treatments in 2014, I became acutely aware that the pathological entities just translocated to other hosts, which seemingly made my treatment easy and 'successful'. Realiz-ing that pathological entities were not so bothered about changing hosts, I knew that I had to stop treating in this way and to change my usual protocols, as more and more I felt it was unethical to simply translocate the disease. Then came the crucial and import-ant moment (in March 2014) when I made the *intention* and came to a clear *desire to stop* this translocation. At the same moment, the effectiveness of my cancer-treatment more or less stopped. The curative effect of my cancer treatment was halted not only for me, but also for most of my students. This happened simultaneously, without anyone knowing of anyone else's experiences.

Since 2014, I have been working to restore the effect of my treatment without translocating the disease. Finally, in 2017, I began making headway towards a solution to this dilemma.

It is of crucial importance here for us to discuss, describe and understand the treatment protocols that one can use to

---

*One may argue that to cause a translocation through treatment will cause no more suffering than if the illness were translocated from a person in the 'normal' way. However, we should bear in mind that an actual *transformation* will, in the long run, create a diminution of the demonic presence in the world. We owe it to the world, as therapists, to lessen the total presence of the adversarial forces.

enable transformation, and the resultant true annihilation of disease.

As written earlier in this book, the bulk of all internal diseases in animals originate from the owner. This phenomenon has also been described in many ancient texts such as the Bible. Therefore, once it becomes clear that the owner is translocating his disease to the animal, child or other less-dominant human, it becomes necessary to treat both the 'alpha-human' (the animal's owner, the parent, spouse or partner), in order truly to transform the pathology in its entirety.

For example, I treated a woman with anxiety disorder and found that, a few days later, her dog stopped urinating in the house. This happened without directly treating the animal and therefore represented a truly transformative treatment for both of them. I have relayed this information in my courses, and the feedback from my students and colleagues has substantiated this finding. Additionally, translocation can occur amongst the members of a household. For example, I have seen chronic cystitis in a female patient, only to observe the same pulse pathology and translocated prostatitis in her husband a few months later. However, by treating the wife and husband through transformational techniques, both were cured. Without using the methods that facilitate transformation (a *cure*), we resort to accomplishing only one of three things:

- First, we can merely *palliate* the case, as we watch its repeated return months or years later.
- Secondly, we can *suppress* the disease by substituting a less sinister pathology with a much worse one.
- Thirdly, we can translocate the disease to another entity altogether.

An example of the second possibility is the use of steroids to suppress an atopic dermatitis, only to replace it with, for example, Cushing's disease later.

If one reviews the literature of various alternative medical systems, there are revelations that show that this translocation phenomenon was being observed in earlier times, especially by some of the great physicians of homeopathy, such as Dr Constantine Hering, the founder of 'Hering's Law of Cure'. The gold standard of the evidence of a cure was eloquently categorized by this physician as a centrifugal exteriorization of the symptoms, from serious spiritual and organic disease to superficial areas such as the skin – the eventual positive outcome being a person with total freedom of body, mind and spirit in order to enlist his higher calling. What was not overtly addressed in this law was the transmission of such demons to other beings on the planet. Therefore, from a global perspective, this does not represent a cure.

For the last 30 years, as both an anthroposophist, a veterinarian and an acupuncturist, I have tried to find methods of treatment that do not merely translocate, palliate or suppress the pathology, but rather result in a transformation in order to evoke a truly curative response. During my search, I gradually discovered that each 'acupuncture technique' I modified resulted in different effects on my patients, as shown below:

- *5-element* system of Chinese acupuncture, where translocation seems to dominate.
- *6-element* method, where suppression seems to dominate.
- *7-element* method, where transformation seems to dominate.
- *12-element* method:
    - in a star-pattern, relating to the zodiac: here both efficiency and transformation seem to dominate in eighty per cent of patients;
    - in a 90^0-controlling pattern (based on knowledge of morning and midday forces, explained on p. 63.) both efficiency and transformation seem to dominate in close to one hundred per cent of all patients.
- *Middle Point in a single patient*: the spiritual disease resolves but the physical pathology often remains.
- *Middle Point in a circle of patients*: higher spiritual beings are enlisted and seem to help create a deeper and more karmic spiritual healing amongst the entire group, but physical pathology often remains.

Numerology

It is important to note the significance of *numerology* in treatment. I have come to realize that there is a strong correlation between the numbers of the paradigm and the spiritual structure of the society from which they emerged.

For example:

- The number four was emphasized by the Greeks, the society that embraced freedom, as the elements of Water, Air, Earth and Fire.
- In contrast, the more patriarchal and class-structures of the Chinese adopted a more organized and controlled 5-element system, which not only added the element 'wood', but placed it in a generating and destructive sequence.
- The importance of a trinity was embraced by the Tibetans.
- The more sinister number six was emphasized by Yahweh, the merciless Moon god, and Islam.
- As an anthroposophist representing the work of Rudolf Steiner, I have found much of interest and truth in the significance of the number seven. Steiner described the significance of this number in advancing the spiritual evolution of mankind.
- The number twelve mirrors the number of zodiacal signs, and as such encompasses the whole of the cosmos. It also expresses the number of the disciples around Jesus Christ, the truest transformational force known.

The choice of the system we decide on will therefore influence the results of our therapy, whether it will be a suppression, a translocation or a true transformation.

Learning How to Treat Cancer

Sometimes, our greatest struggles guide us to our greatest achievements. For me, this struggle came with the treatment of cancer. The dilemma began with my use of acupuncture meridian therapy according to the 5-elements.[43]

As mentioned above, my journey towards understanding the nature of cancer began in the 1980s. I realized at that time that cancer had to be treated differently from other disease processes. The solution seemed both simple and profound. Using the principles of 5-element acupuncture, I saw cancer as simply an excess of a normal fundamental process. Therefore, the meridian organ system controlling that process must be deficient. My conclusion was to strengthen the deficient system and to regain control over the excess. I called this method: 'the controlling treatment'. I believed at that time that this was a superior method to treating the excess directly, which represented the Western medical modality of suppressing the growth of the tumour through surgery and chemotherapy. I was under the misguided belief that this might hold the key to curing cancer in the future.

For several years, the results seemed to prove my theory. In 1984, I first applied a 'controlling' treatment method on a dachshund. The dog had multiple tumours along the mammary chain and was struggling to breath, indicative of pulmonary metastasis. Using acupuncture, I treated a strengthening point on the liver meridian (liver 03 – LR03), in order to tonify this meridian/organ system. As the liver controls the stomach meridian (the residence of the mammary chain), such a treatment should take control of the cancer. In a few weeks, the tumours disappeared completely. The dog died several years later of old age (from renal failure).

Another example of this successful protocol occurred in 1995, when I used this method for the first time to treat a horse with cancer. The horse was diagnosed with an equine sarcoid, a form of skin cancer. The result was promising, as the sarcoid disappeared within six weeks.

Between 1984 and 2014, I treated more than one thousand animal and human patients that were suffering from all kinds of cancer. The results were especially good with mammary cancer (85%), and in melanoma (80%). The results in lymphosarcoma and brain cancer were moderately good (70%). However, my results with liver and pancreatic cancer were mediocre; the healing rate being 'only' 60% in the few patients I treated.

My success with treating cancer patients using the 5-element controlling method continued for thirty years, up until 2014. I then *understood, intended* and *decided* to try to stop translocation. This mere wilful *decision* triggered a huge response from the pathological entities. They sensed the looming disaster of transformation (demons seem to fear it). I began to notice a resistance to the 5-element treatment. Although the tumours would still shrink, the actual ability to cure the patient declined. After some months, the effect had totally disappeared. To make matters even more confusing, my closest students were experiencing the same phenomena. The only ones that were still having some success where those physicians that had learned the method from my writings, rather than through me directly. The efficacy of the controlling method on treating cancer continued to decline throughout 2014, until it was close to non-existent. I was baffled by this change in events.

I did not despair, but worked hard to find out the reason why the effect had vanished, and to find a better method.

The Middle Point, a New Concept of Treatment

In 2016, I understood clearly that I could not use acupuncture according to the 5-elements to treat cancer. I then decided to try employing *Christ Consciousness*. I discovered this point by studying the works of Judith von Halle.[44] She states that a diseased patient should be healed using 'Christ Consciousness'.

I was still in confusion: How do I treat with Christ Consciousness? After looking carefully at the wooden sculpture made by Rudolf Steiner and Edith Maryon called 'The Group' or 'The Representative of Man' – which depicts Christ standing between the two dominating adversary and pathological entities, Lucifer and Ahriman – I realized that the healthy energy of Christ Consciousness lies between these yin and yang structures residing in the body. I named the loci that could accomplish this task the 'Middle Point'. Using this point, I treat neither the excess nor the deficiency, but try to stimulate the Middle or healthy area that lies between these two opposites.

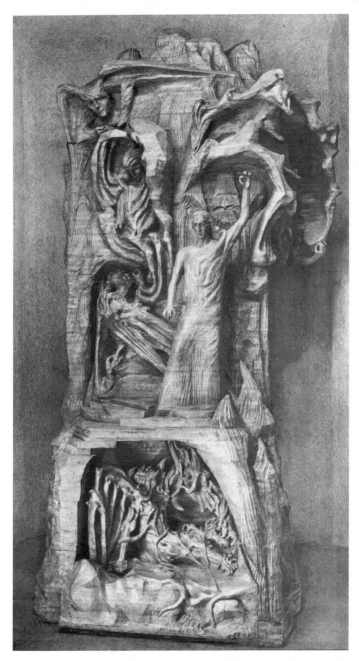

*Rudolf Steiner's 'Group' sculpture made with Edith Maryon, showing Christ
between Lucifer (above) and Ahriman (below)*

The first time I attempted to treat the Middle Point was on a horse during a veterinary course in Germany. I clearly saw, with my spiritual eyes, a 'yin-pathological structure' (the ahrimanic double or demonic structure) in the region of the abdomen, and a 'yang-pathological structure' (the luciferic double or demonic structure) in the region of the upper chest and head area.[45] Using my spiritual vision, I could also locate the Middle Point. The following 'treatment' of the Middle Point (or, one could say, its activation and subsequent separation of both adversary forces), resulted in a remarkable healing of the horse.

I realized that these adversarial upper and lower (cranial and caudal) structures have a kind of life-force of their own and, as such, require the gentler treatment of an acupuncture needle, or even one's fingers. In contrast, a dermojet[46] forces fluid into the point by a forceful thrust of pressurized air. Electrical stimulators, magnetic wave generators and cold lasers are also ineffective and can be detrimental in treating the Middle Point (the Christ point). This is due to the fact that the adversarial entities thrive on these types of devices. Since 2014, I have treated many human and veterinary patients using the Middle Point – that is, as single patients and not in a group, as will be discussed later – using one needle carefully placed in the Middle. Alternatively, with my fingers held in the gesture that Christ makes in the 'Group' statue, *pushing the luciferic and the ahrimanic entities apart, and making way for the Christ-force to enter.*

Most patients seem to be satisfied with the effect of this treatment, although the medical results appear to be less than the spiritual effect. This means that the healing takes place through the higher spiritual sheaths of the patient, and not directly through the etheric or physical body. Some patients describe an intense feeling of healing energy radiating throughout their bodies. I can see patterns in the shape of a figure eight combined with a spiral streaming in.

I discovered that using the Middle Point does not necessarily heal the physical disease itself, but rather activates a more spiritual kind of healing, which then often also heals the physical disease. This is also the case when activating the Middle Point in a group situation, that is, treating several patients gathered together, sitting in a circle.

Later I discovered that by combining the treatment of the Middle with a non-translocating healing method (see later the 7-element method or especially the 12-element method), will initiate a curative response by healing both the material and the spiritual aspects of the patient.

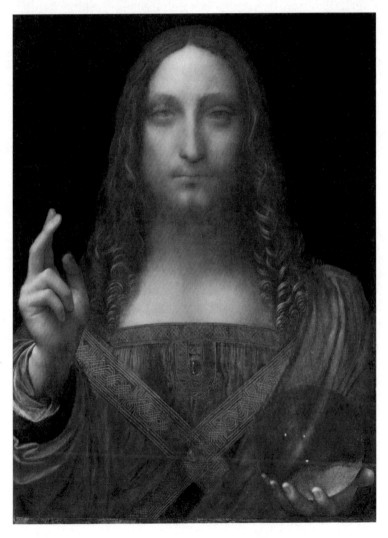

Salvador Mundi by Leonardo da Vinci

The above painting illustrates in a perfect manner the placement, structure and importance of the Middle. The Middle is situated just between the luciferic forces and the ahrimanic forces in the body, in the area of the heart. If the disease is not caused by translocation of a demonic entity from outside, but is due to an excessive presence of either the luciferic or the ahrimanic forces within the body, we should put these forces back into the preferred and correct position. It is important to remember that these forces are necessary for our very material existence; without them we could not exist in the material world. It is only an imbalance of luciferic or ahrimanic forces that creates disease – and through such an imbalance, individual demons can be released which lead to a creation of diseases in children and animals.

We put the adversarial forces back into their correct position by strengthening the Middle, the Christ-force. This is threefold—it exists in three dimensions. The presence of the adversarial forces is also threefold and exists in three dimensions:

- The luciferic forces are more to the head, to the left and to the front.
- The ahrimanic forces are to be found more towards the pelvis, to the right and to the back.

In this way, we should widen and strengthen the Christ-force in all directions, as a sphere that is enlarged, just as is depicted by Leonardo in the image above.[47]

This Middle can be treated in many ways, but I find the best to be the manual method. I hold my hands in the area of the Middle, imagining it to be like the sphere Christ is holding in the picture by Leonardo, and then enlarge it between my hands. Another way is to place a needle in the centre of the Middle point.

This Middle can be found in three places:

- on the head (as in craniosacral therapy), expressing the Christ-force in *thinking*;
- in the area of the chest, expressing the Christ-force in *feeling*; and
- in the area of the abdomen, expressing the Christ-force in the *will*.

There are several ways to find this Middle:

1. Seeing the Middle Point (clairvoyance)

The ability to 'see' the spiritual world can be a natural gift or it can be learned through dedication. For me, it was a skill that I possessed since birth. In my early youth it felt so natural that I assumed that everyone had this ability.

Although I use the word 'see', this does not exactly convey the experience, as the physical eyes are not involved. For lack of a better description, this is as close a word I can use to describe the phenomenon. In order to gain access to the spiritual world, it is necessary to be able to excarnate from the material body.[48]

2. Feeling the Middle Point (clairsentience).

This is the ability to receive information through sensing or feeling subtle energy. It is actually one of the more common psychic gifts, often activated without conscious awareness. Loosely translated, it means a 'clear feeling'. Clairsentience can trigger physical sensations such as tingling, a ringing in the ear, or changes in the practitioner's pulse. In extreme cases, one can even feel physical pain.

For some students, using Nogiér's pulse diagnosis to find the Middle Point is a form of effective clairsentience.[49] Nogiér, a French acupuncturist known for the development of auricular acupuncture, used the pulse as a kind of 'geiger counter' to find various pathologies. When a honing device was passed over a testing zone, the practitioner's pulse, taken at the auricular artery, would change in rate or intensity. Using this same concept, one can pass the finger of one hand over the mid-section, while taking the auricular pulse with the other hand and waiting for a change in intensity or frequency.

Others have found that, while performing this procedure, the patient often experiences a change when the practitioner's finger is passed across the Middle Point. Horses are particularly sensitive and can be observed to chew, drop their heads and/or blink and close their eyes.

For many practitioners, the simple act of feeling the area can be informative. Some feel changes in temperature, while others feel a kind of roughness to the skin that, at a physical level, may not be overtly palpable.

3. Smelling the Middle Point: (clairalience)[50]

During the winter of 2017, I was teaching courses on how to find and treat the Middle in both Calgary (Canada) and Florida. In Calgary, I had a student who claimed to have the ability to smell the presence of disease. With that proclamation, she insisted on smelling each patient to find the Middle Point, which she did accurately. I then proceeded to Florida to teach yet another group. Knowing very well that most did not possess the ability spiritually to see the Middle Point, I decided to test the efficacy of clairalience. I began by emptying my lungs of air, and then with one long inhalation I passed my nostrils along the midsection of a canine patient. Much to my surprise, I found a clear change in the odour at the level of the midpoint. At the exact location, the odour changed from a normal dog smell to a more pleasant aroma. Continuing beyond the point, however, revealed a pathological smell, quite distinct from the Middle scent. After interviewing the course participants, I found that more than half were able to distinguish these three odours (normal – pathological – healing). I coined the phrase 'the sniffing diagnostic test' for my new method of finding the Middle Point.

The exact method involves exhaling all the air from the lungs, and with a long and constant inhalation through the nose, moving the head in a steady pace, over the back of the patient. As mentioned, at the exact location the smell changes to a pleasant odour, and immediately cranial or caudal to the Middle, the smell changes to a somewhat more 'physical', dog-like or even pathological smell. I asked the other participants to do this 'sniffing-test', and about sixty per cent of the participants could clearly recognize the three different smells.

How the activation of the Middle Point can be incorporated into existing therapies such as acupuncture, homeopathy, herbal or anthroposophic medicine

To understand how to use a 12-fold division of the organs, meridians and sense organs – in accordance with the zodiacal forces emanating etheric energy from the voids of the entire cosmos – we must take a closer look at the *spiritual forces* emanating from the various constellations. Relating to this task, we can find Rudolf Steiner's words[51] most enlightening:

> And so, just as it is essential for an orthodox professor of biology to have the most powerful microscope available and the most efficient laboratory methods, so, in the future, when science has been spiritualized, it will be of the utmost importance whether certain processes are carried through in the morning or in the evening, or at midday, and whether what has been done in the morning is allowed to be further influenced by an evening activity, or whether the cosmic influences are cut out, paralyzed, from the morning until the evening. Processes of this kind will of necessity come to light and will run their course. Naturally, a great deal of water will have to flow under the bridges before the professional chairs and laboratories, at present organized on purely materialistic lines, are handed over to spiritual scientists, but this replacement must come about if humanity is not to sink into utter decadence. For example, if the question is one of doing good in the immediate future, existing laboratory methods must give way to methods whereby certain processes take place in the morning and are interrupted during the day, so that the cosmic stream passes through them again in the evening and is in turn rhythmically withheld again until morning. So, the processes would take their course: certain cosmic workings would always be interrupted by day, and the cosmic morning and evening processes would be brought in. All sorts of arrangements would be necessary for this. You will realize that if one is not in a position to take any public action about these things, all one can do is to speak of them.

How the Middle can Heal the Adversarial Forces

Below we see a picture of the main healing forces represented by the line between Pisces and Virgo and the opposing or adversarial forces exposing themselves in the line between Sagittarius and Gemini:

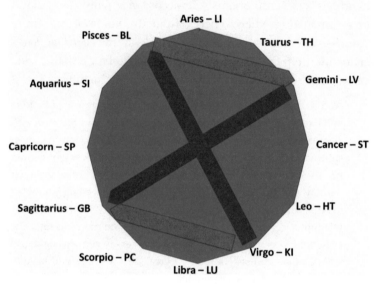

12 elements in transforming cycle

An interesting observation is that the healing forces from Pisces (Christ) can transform the forces of Gemini (Ahriman), and the healing forces of Virgo (Sophia) can heal the adversarial forces of Sagittarius (Lucifer), and that these healing forces arrive in a 90⁰ angle.

Using the Middle Point in a Transformative Way to Treat Noxious Earth Radiation

Earth-Radiation appears to my spiritual eye as black snakes curling and moving along the surface of the Earth. They should not be mistaken for the energetic bonds between trees and plants, which are described in my book *Poplar*. These bonds, although similar in their movement along the forest floor, are much lighter in hue. I have been able to enter these 'tree snakes' with my consciousness, and can 'travel' within this energy pattern.

Travelling in the left direction takes me back in time. I have never attempted to travel to the right for fear of seeing the future. (I consider that the future belongs to much higher powers than my own.) Within the energetic streams of the trees, I have experienced the secret of the 'double stream of time'.[52] The black snakes that are the expression of Earth-radiation are seen as darker and not as transparent as the energy snakes connected to trees. Entering inside the Earth-radiation snakes is not advisable, as they are of a malignant, ahrimanic nature. They represent the past deeds of all humans – the karma of each and every one of us.

This karma of past deeds can either be translocated or transformed; this choice is always ours to make.

- A *translocation* of Earth radiation can be achieved by applying a variety of technical devices, often based on ingenious systems of wires, metals and crystals. As these devices are made and exist in the material world, they usually simply influence the material part of the radiation, whereas the real pathological element is the spiritual part—ahrimanic and/or luciferic elementals 'riding' the radiation.

- A *transformation* of Earth radiation can be achieved by concentrating on the Middle Point within the Earth radiation itself. By this concentration, the strength of the Christ-force residing in the Middle will be strengthened, and the adversarial forces will be pushed back – their cooperation weakened and hindered and, finally, one may hope transformed.

In healing and transforming both Earth-radiation (which is created by humans' ill-deeds in this or in a former life) and electromagnetic radiation (which is created or produced by binding and changing divine elementals, pushing them into sub-nature – which is also a very ill deed), we should – as a fundamental mood in our soul – be asking for forgiveness in the name of Christ.

Using the Middle Point in a Transformative Way to Treat Plants and Trees

For many years I have been able to 'pulse' trees. A German colleague, Ferdinand Niessen, told me he felt that all trees had a weakness in the water element, about one third distal to the top of their structure. I pondered this phenomenon for years until I realized that all humans and animals have a deficiency of water where Lucifer abides, which is the top half of the body. As Lucifer represents heat, we often find a deficient kidney energy in that area. One third proximal to the root of the tree, and one third cranial to the tail base of animals and humans, we can find the ahrimanic influences. Here, there is a deficiency in the 'wood' element, representing the energy and fundamental process of the liver as defined by 5-element acupuncture. Therefore, when we pulse a tree, it is important that we do not pulse the tree one third from the root or one third from the top, otherwise we always get either a deficiency in the liver or in the kidney. This is the same in animals and humans. We have to focus and spiritually enter the heart of the patient in order to get a correct pulse finding. To treat a tree from the Middle Point, we 'needle it mentally' on the Middle Point between the kidney-deficiency and the liver-deficiency, and at the same time 'push' the adversaries back to make more room for the Christ-force. When I do this, I find that both the deficiencies often disappear.

Also, in treating trees this way, we should hold within our souls a feeling of asking for forgiveness in the name of Christ.

Using the Middle Point in a Circle of Humans or Animals

On the evening of 5 November 2016, something unexpected happened. I was giving a veterinary course in New York and, as a demonstration, treated the participants with the Middle Point. Twenty-five human participants were lying on the floor as I needled all the individual midpoints between Lucifer and Ahriman. Then I sat back to watch. The needle that was placed on the thorax, between the adversaries, seemed to activate the area of 'free' etheric force not dominated by Ahriman or Lucifer — the Christ-force.

When this area became activated, a light started to emanate from the chest of the participants, and after a while it rhythmically oscillated. Then, the light started to float up from the participants and began to circle around and over the entire group. This circling became more and more luminous, going upwards in a stream.[53]

What I saw happening within the group was totally different from what happens when I treat an individual. The cooperation of 'the good' in each and every one of the patients was able to transform something into light. The irony of individualized treatment then became apparent. It was obvious that ahrimanic forces are enhanced when man is 'culled from the group'. Sadly, the individualized approach to medical treatment has become the gold standard, especially with regards to immunotherapy. Without an understanding of spiritual science, the medical community is unaware of the power they are giving to the adversarial forces that perpetuate disease.

At the beginning of the twentieth century, Rudolf Steiner predicted that mankind would become increasingly infused with technology. He also believed that this technology would be utilized by the adversaries in order to gain access and control over all aspects of human evolution. He was correct. Mechanization is another means by which ahrimanic forces can fortify their hold on the material world. (This theme is explored in the final chapter.) Once again, it cannot be overstated how, by using the social element of group treatment combined with the absence of machines – using only one single needle in the healthiest point of the body, namely the Christ point – we can go forward in preventing the disastrous cooperation between Lucifer and Ahriman.

Chapter 4

Homeopathy, Western Medicine and Translocation

In this chapter will we will elaborate on the problems, dangers and possibilities of translocation within:

- homeopathy;
- Western medicine;
- anthroposophic medicine.

Homeopathy

I will start by describing homeopathy and how homeopathic remedies are created. This procedure can be instructive for this whole book (especially Chapter 5), as in the making of homeopathic medicines there is a positive translocation in the preparation phase, and often a negative translocation in the therapeutic phase.

Homeopathic concepts and theories have been the subject of discussion, study and trial in most cultures: Chinese, Indian, Persian, American and European. Homeopathy is a very controversial medical modality. The reason for this is the speciality of homeopathic remedies.

- In herbal therapy we give different plants or herbs containing pharmacologically-active substances.
- In acupuncture we stimulate certain points or nerves, which release certain substances or endorphins.
- In homeopathy, from a materialistic viewpoint, we give nothing that can be measured chemically, except the 'vehicle' that carries the potentized remedy.

On standard scientific analysis, the lactose pills that carry the diluted and potentized homeopathic remedies contain *no detectable compounds* except lactose, alcohol and water. The effect of the homeopathic remedy is, then, purely spiritual.

How can it be possible to take the spirit of plants, toxins or metals out of their material foundation and transfer that spirit to an inert remedy?

If this is understood, the following chapter on electromagnetic radiation can become truly clear.

History of Homeopathy

The fundamental principle of homeopathy is found in the sentence *similia similibus curentur* (like cures like). In more precise terms, a homeopathic remedy cures a disease whose symptoms resemble the symptoms evoked in a healthy body, by a toxic dose (even a homeopathic dose) of the agent itself. This principle has been known since antiquity; philosophers and healers like Hippocrates and Paracelsus also expressed the same ideas. The principle comes, of course, from an ancient holistic concept that the symptoms are manifested by the body itself, in order to help an organ or process that is failing to perform properly.

However, Christian Frederick Samuel Hahnemann (1755-1843), a German physician, assembled all the ideas and theories and developed them systematically into a holistic system of therapy. Hahnemann's pioneering book, *The Organon,* is still a key homeopathic reference book today. Hahnemann called this system 'homeopathy' after the Greek words *homoios*, which means 'like' or 'equivalent', and *pathos*, which means 'suffering' or 'malfunction'. (Homeopathy is written in different European languages as *homöopati, homøopati, homöopathie, homopati* or *homeopati.*)

Early in his medical career, Hahnemann knew that the symptoms of intoxication from a substance resembled those that the same substance could cure in very low doses. In other words, when specially prepared in minute doses, the pathogenic substance was made into a remedy. He experimented with lower and lower doses (higher and higher dilutions). During this experimentation with increasing dilutions and his testing of diluted substances, he accidentally discovered the *principle of potentization*. This is that the tincture or substance that we prepare as a remedy must be diluted and *succussed* (potentized) serially, to such a dilution that its concentration eventually approaches zero. At the higher dilutions, the laws of physics would say that there couldn't be a single molecule of the original material remaining in the remedy. Paradoxically, however, and in total contrast to what one might expect from principles of conventional pharmacology, this process potentizes the remedy, i.e. its therapeutic effect becomes clearer, cleaner, more powerful and more exact, as the dilution increases.

Two Examples of Clinical Homeopathy

Late on a Saturday night, a 7-year-old boy grabbed a red-hot poker and threw it on the ground to prevent his granny's carpet from being damaged. In the process, he gave himself a potential third-degree burn, three cms long, on his thumb and index finger. The house was many miles from the nearest pharmacy, and the boy's granny had no anti-burn or analgesic remedies of any kind. However, as it was a farmhouse, there were nettles growing within five metres of the kitchen door. In first-aid homeopathy, *Urtica urens* (common stinging nettle) is recommended for burns. For want of something better to do, the boy's father, a vet, made a crude nettle-extract in tap water. He diluted one drop of nettle juice in a cupful of water, succussed it, and serially repeated the dilution five more times. He gave the boy a spoonful every ten minutes for about an hour. The boy stopped screaming within the first ten seconds of taking the first spoonful. Within two to three days, the lesion had disappeared without a trace. Standard university training would regard this as impossible – the burn should have turned septic and taken two to three weeks to heal. But the clinical outcome was as described – unbelievable! One wonders who would buy expensive analgesics, antihistamines or steroid drugs to treat burns, stings, hives or other skin allergies if all one had to do is find a nettle leaf in the nearest ditch and make a crude, homemade dilution of *Urtica urens* for oral use. However, *Urtica* does not always work as dramatically as in that case.

Many years ago, a worried father brought his little girl to me for treatment. The girl had been struggling to stay alive for the previous two years. At age four, she had drunk concentrated NaOH (sodium hydroxide) and her oesophagus was very badly damaged; it was like dry parchment, lifeless and totally functionless. She had been through countless infections and courses of antibiotics during the two to three years that had elapsed since the accident, and all her food and drink had to be given via an intravenous nasogastric tube. In this case, the cause of the trauma or disease was obvious; it was the corrosive action of the NaOH. I then took some NaOH and potentized it, which means that I made an isopathic remedy from it. She began to take this remedy, five drops twice daily. After just a few days, vitality and function began to return to the oesophagus. After three weeks, the nasogastric tube was removed. After two months, she was able to eat normally again and remained cured. Strictly speaking, this case was an example of the clinical use of *isopathy*, rather than homeopathy.

The Homeopathic Method

Conventional medicine is gradually accepting the therapeutic value of herbal medicine and acupuncture. Unfortunately, however, this is not the case with homeopathy. The reasons for this are multiple, but one of the main reasons is that the remedies, at the usual dilutions, do not contain a single molecule of the initial substance. Another reason is that the clinical effect of homeopathy often *seems to disappear* in double-blind studies. We will consider this in more detail later.

Homeopaths describe what is left in the remedy as the 'information structure of the substance', some kind of 'resonance' or 'hidden information'. Of course, scientifically-minded doctors or researchers find this difficult to grasp or acknowledge. That the vehicle, be it water, alcohol solution or lactose, can carry the information of a plant or metal without one single molecule being present, is in itself incredible. That this 'information' can communicate with the body and induce the body to heal diseases, such as psoriasis, depression or rheumatoid arthritis, is totally absurd to materialistic 'scientific' doctors. And this intellectual riddle does not get any easier when we consider the great amount of time and energy spent on trying to explain how the diluent (an aqueous vehicle) can carry this 'information pattern' – particularly when we consider that some manufacturing methods of homeopathic pills involve the evaporation of the liquid vehicle when the pills are made.

Homeopaths and scientists agree that continuous serial dilution of a substance eventually reduces its physical or chemical concentration to zero. But homeopathic experts claim that succussion (vigorous shaking and striking of the container) between each dilution induces thousands of small bubbles in the vehicle and preserves the 'information pattern' that induces the therapeutic effect of the remedy.

This is where we will part from both materialistic conventional medicine and materialistic alternative medicine. Homeopaths suggest that succussion induces a structural change in the water molecules in the surface tension layer between water and bubbles. In this way, the remedy-free vehicle preserves the information structure or therapeutic signal of the remedy that induces its clinical effect. According to Avogadro's law, the number of molecules in 1 gram of any substance is 6×10^{23}. When we dilute any substance 24 times at 1:10 each time (i.e. D24), the concentration is 1×10^{-24}. Theoretically, there are no molecules left in the solution at that dilution. In practice, it is not possible to detect the substance even at dilutions like D7 or D8. Conventional medicine classes homeopathic remedies above D6 as having no possible toxic effect. At least it cannot reject homeopathic remedies on grounds of toxicity or lack of safety!

From my experiences with spirits, adversarial elementals, demonic structures of luciferic and ahrimanic origin and 'releasing demons', I know that succussion also has an additional effect on the spiritual content of any substance.

I will describe this as follows. For many years I wondered why a remedy had to be shaken so vigorously between each of the stages of potentization.[54] When I began to 'see' the elemental forces in medical plants as well as in diseases, I entered into a deeper understanding of the procedure of making a homeopathic remedy.

The characteristics of the elemental beings within the medical plant used for making the remedy, looks very much like the pathological being that causes the disease. This is the basis of the homeopathic law of *similia similibus curentur*. Homeopaths know or postulate that the energy of the plant or the metal mysteriously translocates into the water when the dilution is shaken. This shaking enables the spirit of the healing plant to enter or translocate into the remedy. This is then called potentiation, i.e., it makes the water 'potent'.

For example, the spiritual effect or activity in arsenic, *arsenicum*, can in homeopathy be divided from the physical substance of arsenic, and thus be used as a medicine, whilst the toxic substance is effectively thrown away.

Of course, this translocated spirit of the medical plant, often called the *demon* of the plant – as the medical plant often is toxic and the plant spirit then often looks very 'demonic' – can further translocate the demon of the disease itself. This is described by Dr Constantin Hering as the law of healing, which of course is the law of translocation.

In the next section on conventional Western (allopathic) medicine, I will compare the effect of the homeopathic remedy to the effect of the conventional medical remedy, and the above will then become clearer.

Allopathic Medicine

We might think that orthodox medicine is free of translocation, but it is not. Translocation in acupuncture, after 5-elements, especially when the excess is addressed, can happen in a matter of seconds or minutes. In herbal medicine, such a translocation may take three days. In homeopathy, it may also take around three days, as the two examples below describe.

In conventional medicine, the translocation usually takes longer – often three weeks or longer – but Western medicine also translocates the disease, just as other alternative methods do.

Example 1

When I was a veterinarian in northern Norway in 1980, I made the following experiment, which I have been thinking about and trying to understand until this day. I wanted to see if homeopathy was as effective as conventional medicine in treating mastitis in cows. I had planned how to do this, and waited patiently for the moment when I was presented with two similar cows in the same barn and with identical mastitis. After some time the opportunity came about, and I put my experiment into action. The two cows stood beside each other, and I treated the left one with conventional medicine (penicillin and sulphur in correct doses), and the right one with pure homeopathy (*argentum metallicum* D6). After three days, one of the cows died whilst the other was 'miraculously' healed. The farmer, who knew about my experiment, was of course convinced that the cow treated with homeopathy had died and that the one treated with penicillin had been cured. He thus wanted me to pay for the dead cow, and he organised a meeting in the barn with himself, the head-veterinarian in the area and me. We were all gathered in the barn as the journals were presented. I was quite nervous, but when the journals were opened it showed that the cow that had died was the one treated 'correctly', whilst the one that was cured was the one treated with homeopathic remedies. Still, it was a mystery why the 'correctly' treated cow had died. After presenting the next example I will discuss why this might be so.

Example 2

Being at a congress of veterinary acupuncture in Poland, I attended a very interesting lecture by a veterinarian on skin diseases in dogs, and how they could be treated by

Chinese herbs. She elaborated at length, and one of her examples was of two dogs with exactly the same pattern of symptoms relating to longstanding eczema. The two dogs lived close by, and one was treated with conventional medicine and the other with Chinese herbs. After three days, the conventionally-treated dog died whilst the other was cured.

The explanation for both these examples is that conventional medicine, herbal medicine and homeopathy translocate the pathological or demonic structure, the luciferic or ahrimanic entities, but at a different speed or rate. Conventional medicine makes the translocation in about three weeks – about the same time it takes for the demon to translocate from a human to a dog that has opened its spiritual sheaths for its master. When treated with so-called energetic medicine, like acupuncture or herbal therapy, the translocation goes much faster – often around three days. In both cows and dogs, the pathological entity translocated to the other animal in three days, and the poor animals treated by conventional medicine got three 'burdens' at the same time: the burden of the conventional medicine itself, the demon that it already had, and the translocated demon from its 'friend'. This was too much to carry, and death resulted.

This shows what intricate problems, moral considerations and difficult situations we take on when we decide to become doctors, veterinarians or any other sort of healer. We then enter a spiritual realm of transformation and translocation, and if we don't fully see all the aspects of this domain – which very few of us really do – we will inevitably make a lot of mistakes and will have to carry much karma on our shoulders.

Anthroposophic Medicine

Although much of the solution to the translocation problem is based on and drawn from the teachings and understandings of anthroposophy and Rudolf Steiner, nevertheless, many anthroposophical doctors do not understand the translocative effects of conventional medicine, homeopathy or other therapies based on directing the therapy against the symptoms – the luciferic excessive symptoms or the ahrimanic deficient symptoms. Many use several of these methods, together with the use of anthroposophical medicines and different therapeutic models, as described in Rudolf Steiner's lectures on medicine.[56]

With the understanding presented in this book, my hope is that all spiritual doctors, veterinarians and therapists will refrain from methods that promote translocation.

Chapter 5

Translocation of Spiritual Forces in Electromagnetic Radiation

This chapter will deal with the splitting of spirit from matter, in:

- homeopathy (as an explanatory part of the following); and
- electricity, as the carrier of ahrimanic beings.

As I will show:

- magnetism is the carrier of luciferic beings;
- electromagnetism is a carrier of both ahrimanic and luciferic beings.

This chapter is an important part of this study, and is in fact the reason why this book came into being. Please bear with the scientific descriptions, as they will be complemented with spiritual-scientific insights.

Our whole society is based on using electricity, and this form of energy is increasingly seen to be a much better option than using coal or gas – due in large part to fears over climate change connected to the burning of fossil fuels. I personally believe that electricity is not the best option, for the reasons given below.

The way electricity is produced is of crucial importance, and actually contrary to what most people would consider to be beneficial. In the production of electricity, natural elementals living in the four elements are converted and imprisoned into sub-nature – into the realm of ahrimanic powers.

The 'higher' the elemental forces that are transformed are, the lower the sub-earthly forces will be. As such, the elemental demonic forces carried by solar panels and nuclear fusion will bring about the worst possible scenario for the emerging Christ-force.

I have observed that:

- Electricity produced from Earth-warmth creates 'gnome-type' demonic beings.
- Electricity produced from water creates 'undine-type' demonic beings.
- Electricity produced from wind creates 'sylph-like' demonic beings.
- Electricity produced from sunlight creates 'salamander-like' demonic beings.
- Electricity produced from nuclear power creates 'azuric-type' demonic beings.

These created demons are 'riding' electricity, magnetism and electromagnetism, as adversarial spirits. However, they can, with the right procedure, be split from their physical component (electricity and electromagnetism are indeed physical and energetic and not spiritual).[56]

To understand this very difficult concept, we will start by repeating the main points of the last chapter.

Homeopaths describe what is left in the remedy as the 'information structure of the substance' – some kind of 'resonance' or hidden information. For example, in homeopathy the spiritual effect or activity in arsenic, *arsenicum*, can be divided from the physical substance of *arsenicum*, and this be used as a medicine, whilst the toxic substance can be thrown away.

If the spiritual part of a substance can be split off from its material foundation, the same effect can also be achieved with electromagnetic radiation (EMR).

First, some definitions and explanations about EMR and Earth-radiation (ER) are necessary. Arthur Firstenberg, in his book *The Invisible Rainbow* (AGB Press 2017), shows and argues that electricity seems to be the main or underlying cause in almost all diseases. Rudolf Steiner suggests that all diseases are caused by ahrimanic and luciferic powers. As electricity is food for the ahrimanic beings, both are correct. Electricity influences us today mainly through electromagnetic radiation (EMR). To understand this complicated concept, we need to know what exactly electricity, magnetism and electromagnetism are.

What is electricity in the eyes of modern science?

The word 'electron', is taken from the Greek word ήλεκτρον, meaning 'light gold', after the colour of amber. From a physical point of view, electricity is in summary a name for all phenomena that are caused by static or moving electric charges associated with electric and magnetic fields. Electricity and magnetism are closely connected and together form electromagnetism, one of the four basic forces in physics known today.

Physical principles of electricity (in the eyes of modern science)

The material carriers of the electric charge today are thought mainly to be negatively-charged electrons and positively-charged protons or ions. Charges of the same type repel each other; opposite charges are attracted. Static or moving electric charges are the sources of the electric field, and moving charges are moreover the cause of magnetic fields. By periodically oscillating the electric charge, electromagnetic waves are excited.

The propagation of the physical part of light in space is associated with such electromagnetic phenomena.

The electric current is based on the movement of electric charges. It is explained in solids by the movement of free electrons, and in liquids and gases by ion motion. In the case of solids, a distinction is made between electrical conductors, non-conductors and semiconductors. The driving force of the electric current is the voltage measured in volts, which corresponds to the potential difference between two points of the electric field.

The smallest quantity of free positive or negative electrical charge is called an elementary charge and is a universal, natural constant.

The Electrical Field

Each electrical charge generates in its vicinity an electrical field, where strength and direction are indicated by the electrical field's strength. It is defined as a vectoral quantity, that indicates the force with which the electrical field acts on a small sample charge at a given location.

Frictional Electricity

Frictional electricity was first found around 550 BC, and was described by Thales of Miletus, who used amber as a tool.

The applied friction force as such has no influence. This results in a separation of electrical charges, which are distributed differently on the materials used. In 1733, Charles du Fay described the two types of charge as 'glass' electricity – which corresponds to the positive charge – and as 'resin' electricity – which corresponds to the negative charge. He also realized that the two types of charge can neutralize each other.

Charles du Fay further says (and this is important for us today):

> You do not know the elementary things of electricity. You know that there is what is called friction electricity, that you bring a glass rod to unfold a force by rubbing it with some kind of rasp or a resin rod. Thereby, the glass rod or the resin rod gets electrically charged, that is, they attract small bodies or shreds of paper. You also know that the observation of the phenomena has gradually revealed that in their unfolding are the two forces which emanate in one case from the grated glass rod, in the other case from the grated resin rod or sealing wax rod. Therefore, one distinguishes the qualitative glass electricity and resin electricity, or by merely generally expressing positive electricity and negative electricity. The glass electricity would be the positive, the resin electricity the negative.
>
> Now the peculiar thing is that positive electricity always attracts negative electricity in a certain way [...] so we see that the forces of electricity that face each other have a certain tension and strive for balance. The attempt will often have been made in front of you.[57]

Contact Electricity

The term contact electricity was coined by Alessandro Volta and stood in contrast to the thesis of animal electricity represented by Luigi Galvani. In fact, 'touch electricity' comprises a very wide range of different electrical phenomena occurring at the interface of contacting substances or at the interface with the environment. Friction electricity is in this sense a special case of contact electricity.

Electricity in Nature

In nature, electricity is most directly and spectacularly manifested in the appearance of lightning. In animated beings, electrical phenomena are connected with nervous and muscular activity. Some fish, such as the echinoderm and the eel, can generate high voltages of up to a few hundred volts and can deliver surges of up to a few amperes.

Magnetism

The word magnetism derives from the Greek word λίθος μάγνης (stone from Magnesia). Magnetism is a physical phenomenon that manifests itself by a certain force between magnets, magnetizable substances or moving electric charges. The force is represented by a magnetic field, whereby the density and orientation of the field lines illustrate the strength and direction of the acting force. In 1820, the Danish physicist and chemist Hans Christian Ørsted happened to observe during a lecture how a wire fed by an electric current deflected a compass needle. In 1831, Michael Faraday discovered the principle of electromagnetic induction, according to which a moving permanent magnet in a wire loop excites an electrical current.

It now becomes very clear that electricity and magnetism are closely linked. As electromagnetism, they form one of the four fundamental forces of physics known today. From 1861 to 1864, James Clerk Maxwell formulated the theoretical foundations of electromagnetism with the Maxwell equations named after him.

What is Magnetism in the Eyes of Modern Science?

Magnetism is one aspect of the combined electromagnetic force. It refers to the physical phenomena arising from the force caused by magnets – objects that produce fields that attract or repel other objects. The motion of electrically-charged particles gives rise to magnetism. The force acting on an electrically-charged particle in a magnetic field depends on the magnitude of the charge, the velocity of the particle and the strength of the magnetic field.

All materials experience emagnetism, some more strongly than others. Permanent magnets, made from materials such as iron, produce the strongest effects, known as ferromagnetism. With rare exceptions, this is the only form of magnetism strong enough to be felt by people.

Opposites Attract (in the Eyes of Modern Science)

Magnetic fields are generated by rotating electric charges. All electrons have a property of angular momentum, or spin. Most electrons tend to form pairs in which one of them is 'spin up' and the other is 'spin down'. Two electrons cannot occupy the same energy state at the same time, so their magnetic fields go in opposite directions. They should then cancel each other out. However, some atoms contain one or more unpaired electrons whose spin can produce a directional magnetic field. The direction of their spin determines the direction of the magnetic field. When a significant majority of unpaired electrons are aligned with their spins in the same direction, they combine to produce a magnetic field that is strong enough to be felt on a macroscopic scale.

Magnetic field sources are dipolar, having a north and south magnetic pole. Opposite poles (N and S) attract, and like poles (N and N, or S and S) repel.

The Earth itself is a giant magnet. The magnetic field is created by circulating electric currents within the molten metallic core.

My 'unscientific' conclusions are as follows:

- Lucifer travels with the magnetic forces, and is fed by electricity (Ahriman).
- Ahriman travels with the electric forces, and is fed by magnetism (Lucifer).

Electromagnetic Radiation (Also From The Perspective of Modern Science)

Referring to cancer in humans chronically exposed to strong electrical fields, the National Cancer Institute, USA, stated on 27 May 2016:

> Numerous epidemiologic studies and comprehensive reviews of the scientific literature have evaluated possible associations between exposure to non-ionizing EMFs and risk of cancer in children (12-14). (Magnetic fields are the component of non-ionizing EMFs that are usually studied in relation to their possible health effects.) Most of the research has focused on leukemia and brain tumors, the two most common cancers in children. Studies have examined associations of these cancers with living near power lines, with magnetic fields in the home, and with exposure of parents to high levels of magnetic fields in the workplace. No consistent evidence for an association between any source of non-ionizing EMF and cancer has been found.[58]

The above statement must be viewed with great scepticism. No government will admit that EMR, especially those caused by power lines, can be the cause of cancer. This is because modern industry depends totally on electric power. Without electric power, mass unemployment, social unrest and anarchy would destroy the economies and social cohesion of modern societies.

Brain Tumors and Exposure to Electrical Fields

A colleague living in Ireland e-mailed me with this information:

> Some years ago, death rate from cancer in workers in a large national research institute was noted to be far above that in the general population. The institute had several laboratories in different parts of Ireland. An investigation was conducted to determine if the deaths could be work-related. The team included a medical doctor who specialized in environmental medicine and Trade Union representatives from each of the labs involved. I was one of the investigators. Exposure to lab reagents, gases,

chemicals, carcinogens, nuclear materials etc. was examined. We could not find a satisfactory reason to explain the abnormal death rate. In one lab, two genetically unrelated scientists had died within a short interval of each other. The cause of death in both cases was a rare brain tumor. Both men worked in adjoining offices. The fuse-box for the lab's power supply was just outside the wall of one office and multiple power cables from that fuse-box ran directly over the heads of both men. The doctor discounted any causality between the cancer in both men and exposure to an electrical field from the cables over their heads. Though I am an experienced researcher and veterinary clinician, not qualified in human medicine, I disagree with his medical verdict. I am convinced that my colleagues died due to cancer triggered by EMR emitted by the power cables.

When a wire is moved in a magnetic field, the field induces a current in the wire. Conversely, a magnetic field is produced by an electric charge in motion. This is in accordance with Faraday's Law of Induction, which is the basis for electromagnets, electric motors and generators. A charge moving in a straight line, as through a straight wire, generates a magnetic field that spirals around the wire. When that wire is formed into a loop, the field becomes a doughnut shape, or a torus.

In some applications, direct current is used to produce a constant field in one direction that can be switched on and off with the current. This field can then deflect a movable iron lever, causing an audible click. This is the basis for the telegraph, invented in the 1830s by Samuel F. B. Morse, which allowed for long-distance communication over wires using a binary code based on long- and short-duration pulses.

Using Will, The Christ Force and The Middle Point to Fight The Malevolent Effects of Electromagnetic Radiation

One may use *will* in fighting the adversaries created by both electricity and electromagnetic radiation. This I will explain below.

The spiritual reality behind EMR

Like everything else in the created universe, the phenomenon of EMR consists of a *material part* and a *spiritual part*:

- In the *material* world, particles and waves will also be considered as material, including the term 'energy', which is also used in many 'alternative' movements.
- The *spiritual* part is not the actual EMR itself, but the spirit beings that follow this radiation.

As we have seen, these are the ahrimanic and luciferic beings, and these beings ride within the hollowness of electricity and magnetism.

The ethers of the divine world may be many- or multi-dimensional, but when the ethers are forced down in the sub-natural world, they lose their multidimensionality and become polar, with a hollow in the middle. This hollowness shows the absence of the divine, and it is here that we can introduce the Christ-force.

When electricity is created, it forms elementary beings of an ahrimanic nature, and when we produce EMR via electricity, we also create luciferic elemental spirits, due to the magnetic part of this radiation.

Electricity is the fallen light-ether and magnetism is the fallen chemical-ether, both of which can be categorized as fallen spiritual forces that are then referred to as sub-natural demonic elementals.

These divine ethers (light and chemical) thus fall into the powers of sub-nature, and as a result 'malicious' elemental beings are created. There are different degrees of malevolence depending on if the electricity is generated from:

- earth warmth (geothermal);
- coal;
- hydropower;
- wind power (wind turbines);
- wave power;
- solar power (solar panels).

The elementals created from these various sources look quite different and they also have contrasting pathological and social effects. Some of the worst and most pathological elemental beings are formed when solar panels are used in the production of electricity. This is logical when we consider that something as sacred as light is being pushed into the sub-natural creation of electricity. It becomes like a double degradation of light.

The pathological and malevolent effects from *electromagnetic radiation* are caused by the adversarial forces 'riding' the electromagnetic wave – from which they can be separated. Then the pathological effect of the electromagnetic radiation will disappear, hypersensitivity will vanish, and we can use electricity as before. We must understand that these adversarial forces come from the *production of the electricity*, and cannot be transformed at the present time. We can fairly easily translocate these forces or choose to try and *transform* them.

- If the electricity comes from a method of production based on earthly forces such as fossil fuels, we will have to deal with the transformed elementals of the Earth, the demonic gnomes.
- If the electricity comes from a production method based on water forces like waterfalls, waves or tides, we will have to deal with the transformed elementals of the water, the demonic undines.
- If the electricity comes from a production method based on wind forces as with wind turbines, we will have to deal with the transformed elementals of the wind, the demonic sylphs.
- If the electricity comes from a production method based on light forces such as solar panels, we will have to deal with the transformed elementals of the light, the demonic salamanders (and they are some of the worst to deal with).
- If the electricity comes from atomic nuclear plants, we will have to deal with the transformed elementals of the Azuras.[59]
- If the electricity comes from a production method based on etheric forces, we will have to deal with the transformed

elementals of the human being, the ahrimanic double. It is therefore of vital importance that we find another source of energy, without harnessing the destructive power of electricity.

An experience in Germany

With this knowledge of EMR, I did the following experiment. At stables in Germany there were fourteen horses, all of which were lame to varying degrees. However, all of them had pain in the spleen area between the sixteenth and the eighteenth rib at the back, and this pain had caused the different types of lameness.

Just one hundred metres from the stable there was a G4 mast. The EMR radiation from this mast could be felt very strongly, and it was obvious that this EMR was making the horses sick. I had gathered a group of twelve people, and at a distance of approximately fifty metres we all attempted to mentally push apart the forces of the adversaries abiding in the mast, and thereby create a space for the Middle Point, the Christ-force. After ten minutes all the pain in the backs of the horses was gone, and within a few days all of them were free of lameness.

I checked the situation two years later and everything was still fine within the stable. The pathological aspect of the radiation was gone, although the mobile phones still worked. The spiritual was separated from the material. This treatment was done by people that did not 'see' the spiritual elementary beings.

An example from the United States

I experienced a similar instance in the United States. Some colleagues and I sat in a restaurant that was 'rigged up' with about twenty television sets, each showing a separate programme. All who were eating there sat like zombies and just shovelled the food into their mouths whilst their eyes were focused deep into the televisions' emissions.

I related the incidence of the horse experience in Germany to my colleagues, and then I proceeded to make the following experiment: concentrating on one of the TVs, I separated the ahrimanic and luciferic powers, and almost immediately there was a significant change in the people who were watching this particular TV. Suddenly, they became humanized, taking an interest in the food they were putting in their mouths, becoming alive in their movements, talking together and showing obvious changes in their behaviour. My colleagues observed this change with astonishment.

The Middle Point of Mechanical and Electrical Devices

This subject is of utmost importance, both now and in the years to come. Today, we all are under very severe attack from electromagnetic radiation. This radiation comes from 4G-masts, 5G-masts, cell-phones (mobile phones) and all kinds of electromagnetic devices.

Since I discovered the Middle Point in living humans and animals, I have for several years tried to find the Middle Point also in 'dead' man-made devices. Contrary to belief that these devices are 'dead', they are creations of the human mind, and are thus endowed with a form of elemental life. They also contain the elemental forces of the luciferic and the ahrimanic realm, without which material existence would not be possible. They also contain the Midpoint, the Christ-point, between the two forces.

I have tried, with 4G-masts, with TV-sets and with cell-phones, to concentrate my will and intentional mind on the Middle Point of these devices, expanding this Middle Point and thus weakening the adversarial forces. Using this kind of 'treatment', I have observed a marked effect on the allergic pathologies of both people and animals affected by EMR-radiation.[60]

Sensitivity coming from EM-devices, the 'allergic' reactions to radiation and the resulting physical pain, have completely disappeared after such a concentrated effort – after such a 'treatment' of only ten minutes. How can this be possible?

If we think about the making of homeopathic remedies, to a certain extent we 'split' the physical remedy from the 'spiritual' remedy, and use the spiritual part as the medical remedy, without having to care about the toxic effects of the material substance.

It is, then, also possible to 'split' the toxic part of the radiation from the devices described – the part that belongs to the adversaries, to Lucifer and Ahriman – and to just keep the 'functional' part, which are the TV-pictures, the cell-phone conversation or the electrical heating of a house.

In such a partial splitting, we have to use our mind of will, where the divided will is first led down into the Earth and then allowed to rise up again. At the halfway point, it must be met by the intentional thoughts of the mind, and in this meeting of will and intent, a force is created to split the pathological from the physical – at least to such a degree that the pathological effect of the radiation disappears.

To repeat: I consider the Middle to be the only force of reality, our only salvation. Our 'logical' conception of reality – in turning everything into polarities – is for me like being dragged into *maya*; the *maya* of illusion.

The polarities appear to be an expression of this great illusion, whilst the Trinity expresses the reality. It is of vital importance to find this *third* aspect in all uses of electricity, magnetism, nuclear power, cosmic streams or corporeal balances, otherwise the ahrimanic-luciferic forces will dominate. *From polarity to triunity.*

We find the same opposition between duality and triunity in the soul forces of thinking, feeling and will. Within each, we must find the Middle Point, the Middle force of love. If we can then relate to and use this Middle force – this power of *Love* as a fourth stream permeating the cosmos – we will be victorious. We then have a cosmic cross, expressed by the morning-evening-midday-midnight forces. Our only salvation is to add the force of *Love* to the fundamental forces of thinking, feeling and will. That is why the cross is a symbol reflecting the love of Jesus Christ.

Appendix

All of my earlier books are each about a specific aspect of the spiritual world and the experiences I have had there.

- *Poplar* is about the spiritual experiences I had in nature, especially with trees, leading back to early childhood.
- *7-fold Way to Therapy* is about the spiritual experiences I had in developing my therapeutic methods, especially relating to the so-called *First Class Lessons* of Rudolf Steiner, given in 1924.[61]
- *The Forgotten Mysteries of Atlantis* is about the spiritual experiences I had in understanding my personal karma, especially in relation to my work.
- *Alternative Veterinary Medicine* is about the spiritual experiences I had as a veterinarian, in trying to find my way from the materialistic medicine of today towards a more spiritual practice.
- *Demons and Healing* is about the spiritual experiences I had in meeting the demonic entities causing disease and creating misfortune.
- *Spiritual Medicine* is about the spiritual experiences I had resulting in the later development of my therapeutic methods, especially in the finding of the Christ-force that resides in the middle of 'everything', and also in understanding the huge danger and illusionary scam that 5-element acupuncture (Traditional Chinese Medicine or TCM) has led us to.
- *Experiences from the Threshold* is about the experiences I have had in crossing the threshold.

These books are all about one thing: to understand man, nature, plants, animals and medicine from a spiritual world view. By 'spiritual world view' I mean a world view based on the existence of spirits. Spirits are 'behind' and are fundamental to all material existence: to plants, animals and man; yes, to the whole Earth. The spiritual world is also 'behind' all kind of diseases, how they are created and how they spread.

What many 'spiritual' men and women in the physical world call 'energy' or 'energy patterns', are in the spiritual world spirits; spiritual entities with a consciousness, an intent, an agenda and an intelligence.

To be able to write the books referred to here, I first had to cross the 'threshold' to the spiritual world. The techniques I have used to do so I call 'translocation' of spiritual parts of my total spiritual composition.

To write the medical books and to practice my way of medicine, I have to understand and to be able to either translocate or transform the spiritual entities causing disease – the demonic forces. Translocation and transformation are thus central in all my work, actions and understanding:

- *Translocation* as the cause of disease and of spiritual movability and initiation.
- *Transformation* as the cause of healing and spiritual development.

In my book *Spiritual Medicine,* I explain the spiritual foundations of my therapeutic methods, especially related to the Christ-force. To use this Christ-force enables us to 'transform' and not just 'translocate' the adversarial forces causing disease and hindering Christ, namely the ahrimanic, azuric and the luciferic forces.

As a scientifically-trained veterinarian and health care professional, I realize that this book will be controversial. However, I would like to ask the reader to suspend judgement and take the opportunity to enter through a door to a world that is as valid to me as the physical world is to all of us. I accept the things that I tell of here because for me these things have always been as commonplace as the book you are reading, or the chair you are sitting upon.

My hope is that this book will be able to reach and appeal to a larger audience than those vested in material medicine. I believe that this information is critical for all who care for suffering and sick humans and animals, from the ravages of chronic disease, and for those of us trying our best to help them. Therefore, I will attempt to present a clear and straightforward picture of what is really happening beyond the veiled existence of the material world, in as honest and personal way as I can.

Notes

1 Concerning the blood of Christ-Jesus on the cross, this matter is much more complicated, but in a way one might say that Christ 'translocated' all sins of the world into his blood, his 'I-am', and as the blood flowed on Golgotha and into the Earth, Christ became the Lord of the Earth and also the Lord of Karma through containing all our sins inscribed in the Earth, later radiating out from the Earth as so called 'Earth-radiation'.

2 See my *Experiences From the Threshold and Beyond*, Temple Lodge 2019.

3 *The Light Course*, GA 320, a series of 11 lectures given in Stuttgart for teachers in the Waldorf-school. The series started on 23 December 1919, ending on 3 January 1920.

4 Most of the acupuncture philosophy and practice is based on the 5-element theory and the conception of yin/yang, and as I often use acupuncture in my treatment, I had the ability to observe these connections.

5 It is very possible that treating a patient according to 5-elements or any other energetic law within acupuncture may balance the energetic forces of the patient; however, this still opens the way for a translocation of the spiritual entity underlying the disease. This is very important to understand.

6 The so called 5-elements can be ordered differently and arranged according to the seven planets and also to the twelve zodiacal signs. This view will as such then correlate more with anthroposophy than Chinese philosophy and thinking.

7 As the 5-element thinking of the Chinese can be transformed or adjusted to both a 7-element and a 12-element thinking, it can also be adopted to a 6-element thinking.

8 Also called the 'deficient' organ in several of my books.

9 Especially *Demons and Healing* and *Experiences from the Threshold and Beyond,* both published by Temple Lodge, 2018 and 2019.

10 Personal communication from the Chinese translator of *Demons and Healing*.

11 Rudolf Steiner (25 February 1861–30 March 1925) was an Austrian philosopher, clairvoyant spiritual researcher and esotericist. As a

highly developed seer, he based his work on direct knowledge and perception of spiritual dimensions. From his spiritual investigations, Steiner provided suggestions for the renewal of many activities, including education (both general and special), agriculture, medicine, economics, architecture, science, philosophy, religion and the arts. Today there are thousands of schools, clinics, farms and other organizations involved in practical work based on his principles. Steiner wrote more than 30 books and gave over 6,000 lectures across Europe. In 1924 he founded the General Anthroposophical Society, which today has branches throughout the world.

12 Edgar Cayce (1877-1945) has been called the 'sleeping prophet', the 'father of holistic medicine', and was the most documented psychic of the twentieth century. For more than 40 years, Cayce gave psychic 'readings' to thousands of seekers while in an unconscious state, in the process diagnosing illnesses and revealing past incarnations of his clients, as well as giving prophecies.

13 Peter Deunov (with the spiritual name 'Beinsa Deuno') (1864–1944) was a Bulgarian spiritual master and founder of a school of esoteric Christianity called The Universal White Brotherhood. His teachings are set out in approximately 7,000 lectures, given between 1900-1944.

14 24 September 1909.

15 With the concept of sin, I do not refer to 'sinning' as meant in our modern world or society, but the actions that lead to hurting one's own or other people's I-consciousness, astral, etheric or physical body.

16 Luke 8: 41-44.

17 It is important to understand that the luciferic and ahrimanic forces inherent in the human body (as well as in all physical/material phenomena of the entire cosmos) are necessary for the material cosmos to exist. It is when these forces become too strong that imbalance will prevail and the forces become demonic. Therapy aims, then, at balancing these two forces by the help of 'the Middle', i.e. the Christ-force. Specific deeds create luciferic and ahrimanic demons. These can translocate, and have to be transformed by the Christ-force of the Middle.

18 Dr Constantine Hering M.D. (1800-1880) is aptly called 'the father of homoeopathy'. Originally a sceptic, he was convinced of its efficacy after an objective study of its principles. He went on to expound upon the laws of cure.

19 Hering's Law of Cure states:

Cure occurs from above and downwards. It progresses from the head towards the lower trunk, that is to say the head symptoms clear first. With regard to the extremities, cure spreads from shoulder to fingers, or hip to toes.

Cure occurs from within outwards and progresses from more important organs (e.g. liver, endocrine system) to less important organs (e.g. joints). That is to say, the function of vital organs is restored before those less important to life. The end result of this externalization of disease is often the production of 'treatment cutaneous rash'.

Symptoms appear in reverse chronological order. More recent symptoms and pathology will clear before old; the disease 'backtracks' so to speak.

20 When my book *Demons and Healing* (Temple Lodge, 2018), was translated into Chinese, the translator contacted me, telling me this knowledge is actually still valid in China. Many acupuncturists know of the phenomenon of translocation, and some try to make the demon go into plants or stones. She further told that the secrets of the 6-, 7- and 12-elements was partly hidden, partly forbidden and partly unknown in China.

21 There are many more details about this in my book *Spiritual Medicine*.

22 There are many stories and insights from old times and old religions where disease and ailments are looked upon as separate and individualized entities, or energetically self-conscious structures, described as elementals, spirits, demons or devas. Many of us therapists have experienced that if we are too open in acupuncture treatment, the energetic pathological structure may jump over and attack us, i.e. inflict us with the disease itself. We have also seen that such pathological structures may inflict, influence or create disease in creatures connected to the patient. We are all interwoven in an enormous web of energy, a web that connects all living entities in the world, maybe even the whole cosmos. This web is to be seen on the other side of the threshold to the spiritual world. It is called by many names: the Akashic Record, karma or the Matrix. This web is made of energy, but not just lifeless, aimless energy. It is made up of elementals, living etheric beings, created by human minds, our thoughts, feelings and actions. This web is also part of disease, and is influenced when we treat energetically.

23 Akasha is a term for 'æther', in traditional Indian cosmology. The term was adopted in Western occultism and Spiritualism in the late nineteenth century. Theosophy popularized the word Akasha as an adjective, through the use of the term 'Akashic records' or 'Akashic library', referring to an ethereal compendium of all knowledge and history. Ervin László in *Science and the Akashic Field: An Integral Theory of Everything* (2004), based on ideas by Rudolf Steiner, posits 'a field of information' as the substance of the cosmos, which he calls 'Akashic field'.

24 Described in my books *Holistic Veterinary Medicine* and *Poplar*.

25 Earth radiation is 'seen' (at least I see it this way) as snakes traversing the room, or the forest – black and shiny, going from left to right or from right to left. One direction goes from the past to the future and the other direction goes from the future to the past. At a certain level, this energy has the shape of a snake; on a higher level it has the shape of a demon. Before 2014, I saw the demons in the shape of snakes, and mainly as 'Earth-radiation'. Lately, I can see them as demons, clinging to humans, causing diseases and pain, depression or anger. Even death can be seen in this way.

26 For several years I used the method of translocating the Earth-grid – the earth-radiation – because I had not mastered or understood the necessity of transformation instead of translocation. In later years I have seen and understood more and more the importance, and also the effectiveness in healing, of transforming the Earth-radiation, the demonic power of karmic residues. Today I only work with the transformative power of asking for forgiveness, and this power, a truly Christian power, works immediately if done in a 'correct' way. See an example on pp. 21–22.

27 The term 'Edda' applies to the Old Norse Edda and has been adapted to fit the collection of poems known as the *Poetic Edda*, which lacks an original title. Both works were written down in Iceland during the thirteenth century, although they contain material from earlier traditional sources relating back to the Viking Age. These books are the main sources of medieval skaldic tradition in Icelandic and Norse mythology.

28 The Norns in Norse mythology are female beings who rule the destiny of gods and human beings. They correspond roughly to other controllers of humans' destiny, the Fates, elsewhere in European mythology.

29 'The Invisible Man Within Us', lecture held by Rudolf Steiner on 11 February 1923, GA 221.

30 'The Mystery of the Double: Geographic Medicine', St Gallen, 16 November 1917, GA 178. (See *Secret Brotherhoods*, Rudolf Steiner Press 2011.)

31 For the spiritual history of Earth see further in Rudolf Steiner, *Occult Science, An Outline*.

32 GA 93.

33 And it came to pass, when men began to multiply on the face of the Earth, and daughters were born unto them, That the sons of God saw the daughters of men that they were fair; and they took them wives of all which they chose. And the Lord said, My spirit shall not always strive with man, for that he also is flesh: yet his days shall be an hundred and twenty years. There were giants in the Earth in those days; and also after that, when the sons of God came in unto the daughters of men, and they bare children to them, the same became mighty men which were of old, men of renown. And God saw that the wickedness of man was great in the Earth, and that every imagination of the thoughts of his heart was only evil continually. And it repented the Lord that he had made man on the Earth, and it grieved him at his heart. (King James Version)

34 *Edgar Cayce's Atlantis*, Little, Van Auken & Little 2006.

35 Lecture by Rudolf Steiner, 4 July 1924 (GA 237).

36 Lecture given in Frankfurt-am-Main, 2 February 1908, on 'The Group Souls of Animals, Plants and Minerals'.

37 Described in my book *The Forgotten Mysteries of Atlantis*.

38 Rudolf Steiner, 10 November 1910, GA 60.

39 See also Axel Burkart's lecture, Die spirituelle Dimension der Klimalüge – Neues zu Klimawandel Klimadebatte und Klimaschwindel: https://www.youtube.com/watch?v=0vLXjQB0ym4&list=UUfuS-f2VRuxbPQqmpxFGYN8g&index=2

40 In traditional Chinese medicine, the meridian system is a set of twelve major pathways throughout the body through which energy flows. Ting points are the acupressure points above the coronary band of the hooves that relate to the beginning or end of these organ meridians.

41 This discovery was primarily made by seeing with my clairvoyant abilities, that I have worked with and trained from childhood. I have written more about how to train clairvoyance in my books

Poplar, Demons and Healing, Spiritual Medicine, and *Experiences from the Threshold.*

42 As my studies of anthroposophical medicine evolved, I concluded that all chronic diseases in man are perpetuated by the inhabitancy of 'yin-pathological entities' (ahrimanic) and 'yang-pathological entities' (luciferic). These structures reside in separate regions of the body; the 'yang-pathological entities' in the cranial midsection, while the 'yin-pathological entities' reside in the caudal area of the body. I also discovered that the level of health of the patient was directly correlated to the distance between these two structures. In a relatively healthy state, the distance in a person approximates 20 cm, while in an average horse they are separated by as much as 80 cm. The closer the two entities migrate toward each other, the greater the pathology. Most importantly, I have 'seen' that, in cancer, there is a minimal distance between the two, as if they have joined forces. Deductively, I concluded that the effect of these demons is exaggerated by their proximity to one another. As I started to 'see' these structures with my spiritual eyes, I began to understand the importance of translocation in treatment. I realized that most diseases were being treated by addressing one of the two 'pathological entities': either by weakening or opposing the 'yin-pathological entity' (treatment of the deficiency) or by weakening or opposing the 'yang-pathological entities' (treatment of the excess). I also discovered that both of these methods are more or less symptomatic, often just translocating the pathology to other places in the body or to other humans or animals.

43 See my *Holistic and Spiritual Veterinary Medicine,* 2017.

44 Judith von Halle was born 1972 in Berlin and is an architect by profession. Since childhood, she felt herself to be especially bound to Christ. She encountered anthroposophy in 1997 and worked part-time for the German Anthroposophical Society until 2005. From 2001 until 2003 she gave lectures in Rudolf Steiner House in Berlin about esoteric Judaism and the Apocalypse of St John. During Easter 2004, the stigmata of Christ appeared on her. Since that happened, she has only been able to consume water – that is, no solid nourishment.

45 The yang structures are almost always proximal or cranial, in the front and to the left. The yin structures are almost always distal (in animals caudal), at the back and to the right. The Christ Consciousness lies between them. This is discussed in detail in my book *Spiritual Medicine.*

46 A device for injecting fluid without a needle, using high pressure and a very fine spurt.

47 It is of course possible that the creation of the 5-elements method to further or force translocation was not simply evil. To transform an adversarial structure or demon, and thus disease, requires the force and consciousness of Christ, and 5,000 years ago the Christ-force was far from the Earth. The Middle Point of man was also almost certainly different to what it is today. Still, according to my intuition, it was still possible at that time to transform diseases instead of translocating them.

48 See further in my book *Experiences from the Threshold and Beyond.*

49 *Auriculotherapy Manual: Chinese and Western Systems of Ear Acupuncture*, Oleson, Terry, Health Care Alternatives, 2014.

50 Clairalience: ('clair' meaning 'clear' and 'alience' meaning smelling) is the psychic ability to obtain specific psychic information based on the use of the nose. Along with its sister abilities (clairaudience, clairvoyance, claircognizance and clairsentience), it makes up five of the six psychic sense faculties.

51 *Reappearance of Christ in the Etheric*, GA 178, lecture 12, 25 November 1917.

52 The 'double stream of time' is one of the most important secrets we should know of before entering the spiritual world. Time can go either way, both from the future towards the past, and from the past against the future.

53 Later I found that this phenomenon, observed for the first time in New York, was only the first third of the process. As described, the activation of the Middle of a group or circle of human beings leads to a liberation of the free etheric energy of the heart, which then begins to circle for about five minutes. Then the energy starts to move upwards to the cosmos. This usually lasts for five minutes. Next, the whole whirl of energy comes down again and enters each of the participants. After a short silence, it begins to circle again, but this time the whirl of energy goes deeply into the Earth and returns to enter each participant. At this point, 30 or so minutes has passed. Then, again the energy starts to whirl, and this time it goes out into the periphery, from where it returns after five minutes, bringing with it a whole multitude of elemental beings. The total procedure lasts around 50 minutes.

54 If a plant is the basic substance, use 10 grams of plant material and put it into 90 grams of 30% alcohol, and let it steep for about a week.

Strain the mixture and keep 10 grams of the liquid. Mix these 10 grams with 90 grams of water (1:9 ratio substance: water). Put this mixture into a bottle so that the liquid fills 1/2-3/4 of it. Shake the mixture thoroughly for 2.5 to 3 minutes (this is what is called succussion). It is helpful to hit the bottle against some padded surface (Hahnemann used his leather Bible). I use this method, and a book bound in leather is perfect. By shaking vigorously, the spirit (often called 'energy') of the plant, metal or other substances used, translocates ('impregnates') into the water. After shaking, the bottle has to stand still for some minutes. You have now produced the potency D1 (or 1X) of the respective medicine.

55   These lectures are to be found in Steiner's Collected Works, volumes 312-21.

56   In many alternative and New Age-inspired circles, 'energy' is often talked about synonymously with the *spiritual*. This is a great mistake that has several unhappy consequences. Energy is a part of the material/physical world and can be measured with the help of physical instruments, such as electromagnetic radiation. Spiritual beings or forces cannot be measured physically – by any means. They can only be observed physically through their effect on the physical/material realm.

57   Charles-Francois De Cisternay Du Fay, *Caroli de Cisternai Du Fay Versuche Und Abhandlungen Von Der Electricitat* (1745).

58   https://www.cancer.gov/about-cancer/causes-prevention/risk/radiation/electromagnetic-fields-fact-sheet

59   Azuras is the name of the transformed elemental beings that attack the 'I'- consciousness of the human being.

60   One very interesting phenomenon that I have observed lately is that the immediate absence of a negative effect from EMR is followed, around three years later, by a *positive effect*. It seems to me that, after three years, the presence of a Christianized EMR actually works in a *healthy* way to *promote* health.

61   See *The First Class Lessons and Mantras: The Michael School*, Steiner Books.

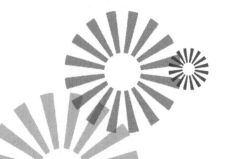

A note from the publisher

For more than a quarter of a century, **Temple Lodge Publishing** has made available new thought, ideas and research in the field of spiritual science.

Anthroposophy, as founded by Rudolf Steiner (1861-1925), is commonly known today through its practical applications, principally in education (Steiner-Waldorf schools) and agriculture (biodynamic food and wine). But behind this outer activity stands the core discipline of spiritual science, which continues to be developed and updated. True science can never be static and anthroposophy is living knowledge.

Our list features some of the best contemporary spiritual-scientific work available today, as well as introductory titles. So, visit us online at **www.templelodge.com** and join our emailing list for news on new titles.

If you feel like supporting our work, you can do so by buying our books or making a direct donation (we are a non-profit/ charitable organisation).

office@templelodge.com

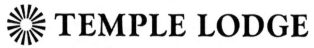

TEMPLE LODGE

For the finest books of Science and Spirit